What Are
We Really Eating?

About this Book

Scientific investigation of nutrition has led to increasing industrialization of food production. Vast numbers of details are known, but industrial processing is causing the force of food to be progressively lost. This makes people feel unsure about which foods are still healthy today.

Otto Wolff's aim is to enable consumers to form their own opinion about the food they eat. He takes guidance from the principle stated by Angelus Silesius: *The bread is not our food; what feeds us in bread is God's eternal word, is spirit and is life*. Dr. Wolff shows that it is not the physical substances as such which feed us but the force of life which is in them. The knowledge that life is transformed light has been completely lost in modern agriculture. But looking at food in the way it is done in biodynamic agriculture can help us gain real insight and understanding of food quality.

This book has been well received, and been translated into many languages, including Russian and Chinese.

About the Author

Dr. Otto Wolff was born in 1921 in Glatz, Silesia (then a region in northeast Germany). He studied biochemistry and medicine and first worked as a hospital physician, then as a general physician and school doctor. Later he worked many years in the pharmaceutical industry in the development of new anthroposophic medicines. He wrote numerous publications on anthroposophic medicine, including the standard work: *The Anthroposophic Approach to Medicine* (three volumes). During his last twenty-five years he taught anthroposophic medicine to medical doctors worldwide. Dr. Wolff died in Arlesheim, Switzerland, in 2003.

Otto Wolff

What Are
We Really Eating?

*Practical Aspects
of Nutrition from the Perspective
of Spiritual Science*

MERCURY PRESS

English language version of *Was essen wir eigentlich? Praktische Gesichtspunkte zur Ernährung auf geisteswissenschaftlicher Grundlage,* 2nd edition, published by Verlag Freies Geistesleben, Stuttgart 2012. (ISBN 3-7725-1244). Revised and amended by Daphne von Boch, MD
and George K. Russell, PhD
Includes additional material by D. v. Boch.
English language edition by A. R. Meuss, FIL, MTA
Edited by Andrea Eberly, MD, Gerald Karnow, MD
Third Edition edited by Peter Luborsky, PhD

Mercury Press
an imprint of SteinerBooks
834 Main Street, PO Box 358
Spencertown, New York 12165
www.steinerbooks.org

Contents

Foreword to the Third Edition 1

Introduction 3

Where Does Life Come From? 10

Raw Food Is 'Sun Food' 16

Can Preservation Maintain Life? 19

Milk and Milk Processing 22

Lactic Acid Fermentation 28

Vitality and Fertility 34

The Role of Vitamins 36

Sugar: Energy Source Without Life 40

The Problem of Food Additives 44

Understanding Digestive Functions 51

      Protein 51

      Fats 54

      Carbohydrates 55

Bread 58

Baking: Archetype of Human Activity on Earth 66

The Problem of Using Yeast in Baking 71

Meat or Vegetarian? 79

Eggs: Concentrated Life 91

The Various Fats and Their Effects 93

Butter 98

Margarine 103

The Cholesterol Problem 110

Future Prospects 117

REFERENCES 120

Foreword to the Third Edition

Today we are in the middle of the problems that this book warned of when it first came out in 1996. The life forces of people, and especially of young people, are getting ever weaker. One can see this in the meteoric rise of conditions such as chronic fatigue syndrome, burnt-out sydrome, repeated infections that last a long time, increasing infertility and the weakening of the immune system. People are getting weaker and more prone to disease, not only physically, but also psychologically. Up to 20% of the patients in medical offices are suffering from depressive disorders—and the trend is rising. A general lack of orientation with respect to the meaning of life is spreading.

What can bring life and light to people again? Things that contain life and light. And this also has to do with food, which should be full of these forces.

In a plausible way, Otto Wolff shows that the important thing for healthy food is not the substances per se, but the forces that these substances contain—and these are life and light. For plants take light from the sun and convert it into life, which is then contained in their substances. When people eat plants, this life and light are liberated inside them. As simple as this thought is, it is very important for practical, everyday life. And this is presented here very clearly through many details and concrete examples.

This newly edited edition retains the changes made in the 2nd edition, in which certain topics were supplemented and others, like the alcohol theme, were added. Since all the new material was based on lectures that the author once gave, his general line of thought has been preserved. Only very few things had to be brought up to date. His witty humor and clear catchy language help to make the reading matter and one's encounter with these ideas stimulating and instructive.

Basel, 2020   *Daphné von Boch, MD*

1

Introduction

Those who begin to think about the food they eat will soon find that there are endless contradictions in this field, more than in any other field of science. It is true, for example, that in civilized countries food is more than abundant in peacetime. Many people therefore believe that our nutrition is better than it has ever been. Others, however, will insist that this only refers to quantity, and that the quality of our food is worse today than it has ever been. Therefore, they say, we should go back to humanity's original nutrition. But what was that nutrition? Some say it was meat, others bread. And what meat and what kind of bread? Some people feel it is self-evident that the only real bread is whole grain bread. Others will actually warn against it and advise eating only white bread, because it does not cause problems with the digestion. Others again advocate life completely without bread or any other grain.

Many people are convinced that only a raw food diet is a healthy diet. After all, they say, animals do not boil or fry their food. Other people will argue that cooking makes the food more digestible and that raw foods are not easily digested. Opposing views are also held on what kind of fat to use. Which is better and which is best avoided—butter or margarine? Opinions continue to clash unabated on many other subjects. It would be easy to give further examples of this kind. The question is, who is right?

Modern people want proof. The situation is difficult, however, because every proponent of an opposite view provides 'proof,' often from personal experience. They say they were sick for years until they changed their nutrition. Since then they have been well. The inevitable conclusion is that if everyone were to eat the way *they* do, all would be well. There is no reason to doubt people's personal experience, but the question is whether others will react in the same way.

There have of course been scientific investigations in the field of nutrition. It has been carefully established how many calories a person needs, how much vitamins, protein, fat, etc. It is important, however, to realize that these investigations can never come to an end. Something 'new' always comes along, which immediately spreads around the world, leaving the 'old' views completely 'out of date.'

When scientific investigation first started, for instance, it was established that only the *starchy* part of grains provides nourishment. The marginal layers cannot be digested and were therefore considered useless roughage. Today, the view is that such roughage is absolutely essential for good digestion. Another example is that just a few years ago, only vegetable fats were considered to be healthy. It was said that all animal fats should be eliminated as far as possible. Since then we have learned that fats from coldwater sea fish such as mackerel have valuable properties and can help to prevent heart attacks. These fish oils are definitely not vegetable fats. And then we often hear that people need specific 'essential amino acids' that are found only in meat, and a vegetarian diet is therefore not sufficient. On the other hand, numerous investigations have shown that vegetarians do not suffer from any deficiencies whatsoever and are undoubtedly healthier in the long run. This is not to say that the scientific findings are wrong! They are, however, often only theoretical or one-sided, and are influenced by other factors that are not so easily grasped in scientific studies.

So what should we do? Try every suggestion? Leave out anything that may be 'questionable?' Mark Twain (1835-1910), the American humorist, already knew about this dilemma. He once wrote that the safest food is water—taken in moderate amounts. Even this is not always true today.

Drinking water is barely drinkable in many places because excessive amounts of chlorine have been added, pesticides or agricultural fertilizers have drained into it, or it has already 'passed' through many people or also through industry. So it is not an absolutely 'safe' food anymore. Even the water 'treatments' used today have their problems. They may remove most of the toxic substances, but they cannot restore the water to its original purpose as the irreplaceable carrier of life.

People who live in arid regions of the world know this very well—without water there is no life. The question is whether the maltreated water available to many people as their only drinking water really can still carry life, compared to fresh spring water. Even the rain falling from the skies has its problems today, as we know from 'acid rain.'

How is anyone to understand all these opposing views and come to an independent judgment? Success stories and scientific findings may be perfectly correct and still miss the point.

These contradictions point to a fundamental problem in today's life. Masses of details are known, we are able to measure and change them, but we fail to recognize the essence of the thing—it is often not even seen. When it comes to nutrition, the essential question is: Why do we need to eat at all? Why do people die if they have no food? Why can we not live only on water, salt, stones or wood?

People had the right instinct in the past when they called food the 'mediator of life' (German *Lebensmittel)*, for it is life that we take in through eating. Stones, wood, or also salt evidently have no life in them, and this is why human beings cannot get life from eating them. Of course there are some exceptions: woodworms, for example, can live on wood; for them wood is a mediator of life, but not for people. So we arrive at a basic principle:

Only what contains life can nourish life.

This may be new to modern people, but it is an old idea. Angelus Silesius (1624-1677) wrote:

The bread is not our food;	*Das Brot ernährt uns nicht;*
what feeds us in the bread	*was uns im Brote speist*
is God's eternal word,	*ist Gottes ewiges Wort,* *
is spirit and is life.	*ist Leben und ist Geist.*

What Angelus Silesius meant is that it is not the physical substance as such which feeds us but its 'content.' It is the force of life that matters—life and spirit.

It must sound truly heretical to modern people to say that we eat God's word and spirit when we eat bread. Do people today know what 'life' or 'spirit' actually are? Those four lines hold more wisdom than the many details we know today. Up to our 'modern' age, everybody knew that food is a gift from God and that it is a sin to simply throw it away. Today this happens with tons of food. Leftovers and waste in the past used to be fed to the pigs or made into compost. They would never have been 'taken off the market'—today's euphemism for the mass destruction of food.

As scientific investigations progressed, the focus was no longer put on life as a force, but on the physical substances. Yet these are only the 'packaging,' for life is not a substance. It is a force, and can only be bound up with certain substances.

As people lost sight of what life really is, they changed their word for 'food' from 'mediator of life' to 'mediator of nourishment' (German *Nahrungsmittel*). There is some justification for this, for not everything we eat contains life. Salt, for instance, does not serve life but higher purposes, as we shall see (see page 47). Roughage, which is really indigestible, also does not contain life and therefore does not nourish us. It does, however, serve the vital functions.

A third group is made up of the stimulants (the German word for these is *Genussmittel*, literally 'mediators of

---

* It is possible that originally the verse had 'light' instead of 'word' here, but that the more common expression 'God's word' seemed more fitting at the time. However, 'light' is clearly more apt. (Author's note) The German word *nicht* ('not') would rhyme with *Licht* ('light'), but does not rhyme with *Wort* ('word'). Ed.

pleasure'), which do not feed us nor help the vital functions. They are only for pleasure, and almost always have a destructive effect on life. The most widely used stimulants are coffee, tea, alcohol, tobacco, and sugar.

Thus, it is *life* that we receive from food. People think today that one cannot really grasp life itself as a force. This is why the declarations on packaging will tell us how many calories are contained in, say, 100 ml of milk. The number of calories tells us how much heat is produced by burning 100 grams of a specific substance. (The more recent term 'joule' is just a different unit of measurement.) This is why we read of the 'calories' or 'energy content' of a food. Useful to a degree, this nevertheless misses the real point. These are terms that are used in the field of technology and have their justification only there. With foods, however, it is not the calories that matter but the life they contain. Gasoline or wax, paraffin and so on, have a very high energy content— high 'calorific value'—but this does not make them food. Listing the amounts of carbohydrate, fat, protein, minerals, vitamins, etc. is a poor solution that does not tell us much, because it does not grasp the essence: life.

Which food has plentiful life in it? Life cannot be measured the way we measure calories. We must therefore start from life itself.

An unborn baby gets its life from its mother. Once it is born, its mother still provides it with milk, which is the ideal form of food for it. From the age of about six months, fruit, grains, cow's milk, and so on are gradually introduced, all of them containing life. Where does the cow get its life from? From its own food, plants, because cows are strict vegetarians. It is very interesting to note that from earliest times people have almost exclusively eaten meat from animals that are not carnivores. We may wonder why. Cows obtain their life from plants; cats, however, obtain their life from mice which themselves are vegetarian. To understand this we have to know that only plants are really able to produce *new* life. Animals get their life from plants. By eating meat from an animal, we take in the animal's life directly, but it comes indirectly from plants. This means that the life which is in an animal is already 'second-hand,' as we might put it today. An animal does not have its life from itself but takes it from the plant, which in turn gets its life from the light of the sun. And 'God's spirit' is in the sun's light, as people knew in earlier times. Life in a plant is much more concentrated. This life is transformed inside an animal, and so becomes available to the animal as *inner* light, as consciousness. Life itself is consumed. If we were to eat the meat of an animal which lives on animals, we would still have food, nourishment, but hardly any more life, because life which originally comes from the sun's light has been gradually reduced in the passage from light $\longrightarrow$ plant $\longrightarrow$ animal $\longrightarrow$ animal $\longrightarrow$ human. This is no theory but has real practical significance. The only possible conclusion must be that a vegetable diet has the greatest vitality.

The graph on the following page shows that even the degree of consciousness of the animal influences the quantity of life in its meat. It shows the amount of food (vegetable substance) in kilograms that a vegetarian animal needs in order to produce one kilogram of meat. Thus, it takes about 9.5 kg of grain to produce 1 kg of beef, but only about 2 kg of grain for 1 kg of chicken. The more consciousness an animal unfolds, the more life is destroyed at the same time. These data are highly informative with regard to feeding the world. If the areas of land needed to grow food for cattle and pigs—both of them bred for food—were instead used to grow grain and vegetables for human consumption, there should be enough to feed the whole world.

Generally speaking, vegetables thus contain considerably more life than meat. The latter does, however, have its own role and justification, and this will be fully discussed later.

We have seen that a plant gets its life from light. It should be possible to free this light again. And this is in fact the case. If one burns a dried plant, then the sun's light and warmth that were in the plant reappear in the fire. Therefore, only formerly alive things that contain light and warmth can be burned. One cannot burn rocks, whereas petroleum can be burnt because it was once alive.

This is not only true in outer nature, but also within animals and human beings. Foods we eat are burned or oxidized in the body, and the warmth that we feel directly comes out of them again. Light now reappears as *inner* light, as consciousness. In the process life is diminished. It is 'consumed,' as we mentioned earlier, and transformed into inner light: into consciousness.

Quantity Fed to Produce One Kilogram of Meat

(kg vegetable substance fed per kg meat)

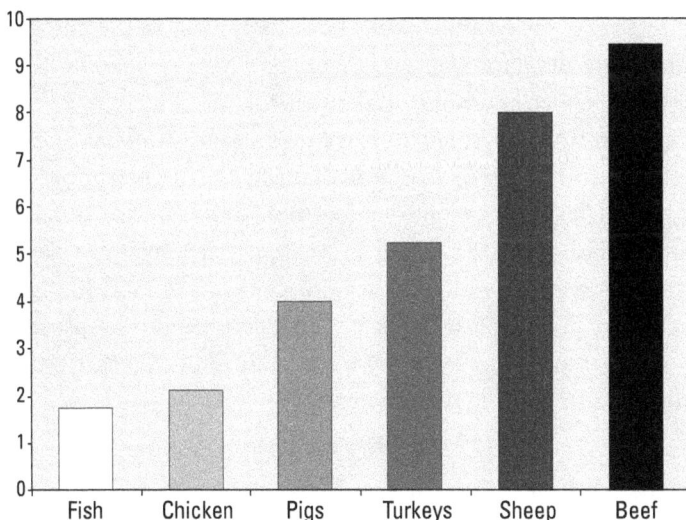

Where Does Life Come From?

As we have seen, cows get their life, their vitality, from plants. This principle applies to all animals, which are therefore called 'heterotrophic,' meaning 'sustaining their life by eating other organisms.' But where do plants get their own life from? Plants are called 'autotrophic,' meaning 'self-feeding.' This is, of course, misleading, as they have to get their life not from themselves but from somewhere else.

Today people are brought up to think that plants 'live' on potassium, phosphorus and nitrogen just as animals live on plants. There is an error in this, however. Animals get their life from the life of plants. Life itself, however, is a force and only bound to physical substance for limited periods of time. Plants cannot take 'life' from substances like potassium, phosphorus and nitrogen because these are completely dead.

Simple observation will show that light is the most important thing for plants. Light is also a force, just as life is. As long as plants are green, they take in light directly. This has been fully investigated. It is known that plants take up light with the help of the green pigment called chlorophyll. They are then able to produce carbohydrates out of water and carbon dioxide taken from the air. Carbohydrates are the substance of which plant bodies are made, and life is active in them. But as soon as light disappears, the plant no longer produces carbohydrates. Life thus comes from *sunlight*. To put it in other words:

Life is transformed light.

Thus, when light falls on something dead, such as a stone, it is converted into warmth. But when it falls on a leaf, it is converted into life.

The question is, why are the above-mentioned minerals important as fertilizers? Life is the most universal force there is. This is why it needs different substances or carriers with which to connect. Water is one of the main carriers of life. 'Living water' is something very different, however. In antiquity people made a very clear distinction between ordinary and living water. Plant sap that is alive, or still alive, contains potassium, for example, because this element 'belongs' to water through every one of its properties. Water has been brought to life in the carbohydrates which the plant produces. The name 'carbohydrate' means 'compound of carbon and water,' which describes it exactly.

Plants need phosphorus as well as potassium to help them work with such substances. Phosphorus does not become part of the live carbohydrate, though without it the plant cannot produce carbohydrates and manage its carbohydrate metabolism. The same applies to nitrogen and protein. (Protein is a compound of nitrogen and carbohydrates.) Certainly no plant consists entirely of carbohydrates. It needs a small amount of protein. However, proteins only gain real significance in animals and humans. Some plants are able to take in nitrogen from the air and can serve as green manure. Otherwise the elimination products of animals have to be used as fertilizers, for they contain nitrogen in organic form.

When plants are given supplemental potassium salts, they are able to take in larger amounts of water. However, this does not increase the level of vitality in the plant. After all, it may only be dead water that the plant takes in together with the potassium. Life is a force, and unlike water, forces cannot be measured in weight. But people think that a greater, heavier quantity of food also means greater food value. The same applies to nitrogen. Organic nitrogen can be taken up from manure, thus maintaining the cycle of life. *Artificial* fertilizer contains nitrogen in the form of nitrate. This is easily soluble and therefore easily taken up into the plant; indeed, the plant is forced to take it up, which may result in nitrate residues. These residues are highly problematic, as they are converted to nitrosamines which are toxic and cause cancer. Thus in a way, the solubility forces the plant to take up these substances. It is another matter if it can process and transform them in the right way for its metabolism. It should be noted that wrongly treated or stored stable manure may be as bad as or even worse than artificial fertilizer.

Thus, fertilizers and manure only provide plants with instruments or aids for producing life from light. Plants cannot take life itself from them. However, the more alive, in other words the more organic the fertilizer (like manure), the more effective it is.

There are ways of approaching 'fertilization' from a completely different angle, and that is through light and life itself. This is the approach farmers use in *biodynamic agriculture*, a method introduced by Rudolf Steiner. Biodynamic products are marketed under the Demeter label. Farmers using this method recognize that plant growth depends not only on sunlight but on the whole cosmos. With insight into individual cosmic factors, which we can certainly have today, we can stimulate plants to be receptive to those influences by using suitable organic preparations. This will strengthen their genuine vital quality. The effect achieved with the use of such preparations is visible. Not only are the plants lighter in color and in better condition, but animal health and the flavor of the products are also improved.

In recent decades the whole food situation has changed because yields per acre have risen enormously. This has been possible through *intensive* farming methods. It has been possible to develop plant and also animal varieties that give better 'yields.' Selective breeding is one-sided breeding that aims mainly to maximize yields and tends to measure easily assessed variables such as gluten and starch content, baking qualities and so on. What is not considered are variables such as life or data from long-term nutritional experiments like those done with milk (see page 25), which can give important information on the real value of the food.

It is important to realize that selective breeding demands high performance which is soon exhausted. New seed must then be bought. This applies to potatoes as well as to other plants, and even animals. What it actually means is that their reproductive strength is exhausted. The life force in them is not strong enough to produce a new plant. The old varieties of grains were undemanding and resistant. Selectively bred new varieties depend on artificial fertilizers and agricultural chemicals as plant 'protectives' to be able to live at all. New varieties are even tested on fields with artificial fertilizers. Plants that do not tolerate them are eliminated. This is perfectly *logical*, for it is the artificial fertilizers which enable selectively bred varieties to give such high yields, but it is not at all *bio*logical thinking.

Selective breeding and artificial fertilizers thus go hand in hand. Maximum yields call for appropriate 'instruments,' such as the application of nitrogen, phosphorus and potassium that we described above. Plants which are not yet specialized for high performance but live in balance with their environment do not need these artificial fertilizers, because a living, cultivated soil with an abundance of different plants produces a harmonious balance by itself.

The same applies to selectively bred cattle, pigs, laying hens and other organic 'producers.' They depend on special feeds. The high performance of a 'modern' cow with a voluminous udder that produces 20 to 25 liters of milk twice a day can only be achieved by feeding concentrates to the animals. It is quite impossible to say where the 'concentrated strength' of these feeds comes from. Statements concerning calorie, joule, protein, vitamin and mineral content, say as little as declarations on milk cartons tell us about the true vitality and the quality of the substances contained in the product. Such data are necessary to a degree, but they miss the point. Basically this is almost as if we were to judge a piece of music only by the volume of sound.

A cow producing such an amount of milk clearly will need extra calcium. It makes a difference, however, where the calcium comes from. Some years ago, people did not hesitate to feed cows for many years with bone powder, together with protein, which the animals also 'need,' both taken from dead animals. The fact that cattle are strict vegetarians was completely ignored. Feeding them animal products derived from cattle themselves went totally against their nature. The animals were forced to be cannibalistic, as it were. This kind of feeding shows that people have completely lost all feeling for the natural needs of a creature. It is based on a purely materialistic way of thinking where only physical substance matters and quality is neglected in favor of yield. These additives finally came to be banned between 1988 and 1990 in different countries, when mad cow disease (BSE) developed, in which the animal's brain is destroyed. It would have been more appropriate to speak of 'mad *human* disease,' for the disease was provoked by 'mad' people. Their madness was the idea that animals or plants should 'produce' like a chemical factory and therefore be treated industrially like chemicals. The cow is looked at like a test tube. If it lacks calcium and protein, they are simply added in, as in organic chemistry. It is of no importance where these substances come from. This is truly madness. It has meant not only incalculable material losses but also great suffering for people and animals. The time has come when it has to be realized that this was not just some kind of industrial accident, but a serious error in the way people think about and relate to nature and to life. Our innate instincts towards nature have clearly been lost, and instead we must now learn to replace them with *knowledge* of the relationships present in nature.

More examples will follow which show that it is not the short-term or most obvious problems with wrong or inadequate feeding that matter, but rather the long-term effects that influence the whole of life. Insight can never be gained by studying ever smaller units such as prions, active principles, genes and so on, but only through knowledge of the essence and meaning of life and nutrition.

It is noteworthy that Rudolf Steiner gave a lecture on the 13th of January 1923[1] in which he said what would happen if an ox, for example, were fed meat. It would 'produce harmful substances' which 'would go to the brain, and the ox would go mad.' That is exactly what happened with mad cow disease.

Raw Food Is "Sun Food"

Fruits are generally eaten raw. But why are potatoes cooked and grain baked into bread? The heat that is used changes the food, breaking it down slightly. Keen advocates of raw food nutrition dislike the idea intensely because something is destroyed and 'lost' in cooking. Considering the matter more closely, however, it looks like this: ripe fruit has been 'cooked' by the sun. The term 'sun food' applies exactly to it. If there is little sun in autumn, grapes will be sour, apples hard, and so on. To put it more exactly, the sun's warmth changes the starch and acids produced in the plant into sugar and aroma that indicate ripeness. The situation varies from plant to plant. Ripening is fast with cherries and strawberries; it is slower with apples, giving them in general better keeping qualities. Every housewife knows that unripe fruit can be made tasty by cooking. Cooking is, in fact, a form of late ripening or predigestion. The ancient Greeks knew this. They used the term *pepsis* for both cooking and digestion.

Suitable heat treatment will thus predigest a food, making digestion easier. It depends on each particular food whether and for how long it should be exposed to heat. People tend to go to extremes. Some will only eat cooked foods, finding them 'more digestible.' However, in the long run this will weaken their digestion. At the other extreme, a diet of nothing but raw food can be a strain, for it involves the whole person too much in the digestive processes. A raw food diet taken for a few weeks (for instance, four weeks) as a treatment can, however, retune the whole organism, something which has often proved effective especially with chronic diseases. In the same way a 'cooked diet' can relieve a weakened organism for a time, which may be helpful, but in the long term will weaken it.

Healthy people therefore do not need to eat only raw foods all the time. A raw food diet is medicinal. It is, however, advisable to eat about one third of the daily food intake raw. It is important to realize that 'raw' should also mean 'fresh.' A six-month-old apple has clearly lost much of its vitality. Dried fruit, even if uncooked, cannot really be called fresh. It hardly needs to be mentioned that 'fresh from the can' is anything but fresh.

The choice between cooked and raw depends primarily on the food in question. Fruit has been 'cooked' in the sun, but not potatoes. Grains, which are fruits, are in a separate category. From early times they have been ground and cooked to make porridge, or more frequently made into bread in a special process which will be discussed later. For some people, however, such preparation may not be strong enough. Thus, it has been found that especially people who tend to develop repeated infections (above all flus, that is, viral infections) or are weak in general (chronically tired, allergic, and so forth) can be helped by eating *raw*-grain muesli.

Raw-grain muesli differs from Bircher muesli in that it is not based on *rolled* oats, which are usually not really fresh, but on *freshly* ground grains which are then eaten raw. These are ground to a fine flour shortly before being eaten. Ideally one takes rye, barley or oats. The vitality of grains depends on their capacity to germinate and on how recently they were ground. After the grinding the grain starts to lose life, but if it is eaten shortly after grinding it still maintains much of its vitality. About two or three tablespoons of the grains are ground to a fine powder each day (not in advance and stored). Soak in water (not milk), ideally overnight, using just enough water to cover the grain. About 8 to 12 hours later, in the morning (or vice versa), the mixture should be sweetened with a mashed banana (no sugar!), which will also make it smoother. Sour milk, sour cream or yogurt should be added (not milk). Fruits of the season may also be added, as well as nuts and sunflower seeds.

Medical evidence has demonstrated that this raw-grain muesli (recipe of Werner Kollath or Max Otto Bruker), if eaten daily for four weeks, will stimulate the immune system. It does, however, require that for this period one must do without sugar and anything containing sugar (chocolate, jam, cake, and so forth). This includes all synthetic and natural sweeteners (honey, raw cane sugar, concentrated agave juice, maple syrup, and so forth). It is acceptable to occasionally eat small amounts of dried fruit, best mixed with nuts, or to drink fresh fruit juices diluted in half a glass of water. All fresh fruit, with the exception of grapes, pineapples and mangoes, can be eaten in unlimited amounts.

Can Preservation Maintain Life?

All plants have their own period of ripening and fruiting. People have always tried to bridge the winter period by storing food. The life of the moment cannot be preserved; the aging process cannot be stopped. It can, however, be slowed down or almost stopped. Probably the oldest method of doing this is *chilling*. The lower the temperature, the more intensive the effect; life becomes frozen. Everyone knows today that this may also destroy cells; they burst through the ice when foods are deep frozen. Fruits that contain much water, like raspberries or apples, can be deep frozen, but when they are thawed they will not be as before. It has also been found that not all vital processes are stopped by the cold. Liver, for example, should not be deep frozen for any length of time, for chemical changes occur even in the deep-frozen state that may actually prove harmful.

Another ancient method of preservation is *drying*. Grass is made into hay for winter feed. Natural drying happens when grain ripens on the ear, which allows it to keep for years. The test for showing that it still has life in it is germination when it is put in water and warmth. However, it is not certain that grain seeds found in Egyptian pyramids were really still able to germinate in our time, 5,000 years later. The reports are contradictory.

Heat will also preserve, not only cold. Through modern scientific investigations it has been shown why living substances will not keep. When an animal is killed, life is withdrawn from its living substance, but this life is not 'gone' all at once. For some time it will still be there to a degree, although the wholeness of the life process, the life-body, has withdrawn from the meat. (If this were not the case, organ transplants would not be possible.)

The same applies to fruits, which tend to continue with their ripening after harvesting. Once ripeness has reached its peak, however, aging begins. This goes on at a different pace for different fruits. As soon as the protective outer skin has been injured or the fruit has been squashed, or when it is mashed and pressed to extract the juice (as with apple juice), alcoholic fermentation rapidly follows. Pasteur's investigations (see page 22) showed that alcoholic fermentation is due to microorganisms called yeasts. When these are killed by heat treatment and the juice is then put in airtight containers, the product will keep. Bottling fruit, vegetables, and meat in jars, bottles and cans is based on this process. Once the containers are opened, letting in air with all the bacteria and yeasts which are in it, rotting or fermentation will begin. The food is broken down further. Thus, canned food still has 'life' in it but evidently not in the same quantity as fresh products. The amount of life which is left will depend on the method of preservation.

Even old, spoiled meat that is no longer fit for human consumption still has life in it. There are creatures that will literally feast on it, among them vultures, rats, flies, maggots and bacteria. They live on such meat; its life is still adequate for creatures which are specialized for this sort of food. Human beings clearly need 'more' life, or a higher quality of it, and this is present when the food is still fresh.

Smoking is another old method of preservation. Smoke contains substances which kill the bacteria that cause rotting. However, it also contains carcinogens, substances that cause cancer. (If smoking were not a well-established traditional method and someone wanted to introduce it today, it would undoubtedly be strictly prohibited because of the danger it poses.)

Also *alcohol kills* germs. *Lactic acid,* on the other hand, only inhibits growth of germs.

Finally *chemicals* may also be used to preserve foods. Some have more or less disinfectant properties that inhibit bacterial or fungal growth for a time. Benzoic acid is an example. It occurs naturally in resin and bark and is frequently used today for short-term preservation.

Milk and Milk Processing

There is only one food in nature which goes straight from one living organism to another. This is milk. Milk differs from one animal species to another. Human milk also has qualities of its own which cannot be found in any animal. This has been discussed in detail elsewhere.[2] Babies take their milk directly from the nursing mother's living organism, which gives them the full forces of life it contains.

This applies to mammals. Human beings, however, take milk from the cow that is intended for the calf. This creates a problem. The milk is intended by nature to be taken immediately and fresh, but only rarely can be consumed that way today. Who has a cow right near their house? Due to bacteria which are present all over in the air, milk will turn sour relatively quickly. Depending on temperature and 'hygiene' it will do so in two to four days. This period can be lengthened today, thanks to the discovery made by Louis Pasteur (1822-1895). He found that certain bacteria which are present everywhere live on the sugar in milk. In the process, the milk sugar (lactose) is changed into lactic acid (lactate). The acid makes the protein coagulate and stops putrefying bacteria from getting into the milk. This results in *sour milk*, a milk which is naturally preserved for a limited period. Lactic acid fermentation can be prevented by killing the lactic acid producing bacteria, which are called lactobacilli. It is done by heating the milk to 70°C, a process known as pasteurization. Milk that is treated like this is labelled *pasteurized milk*. The milk will keep longer, but not for very long, for this method only kills the highly sensitive lactobacilli. It does not kill the more resistant putrefying bacteria. These continue to change the milk protein even after pasteurization, with the result that the milk turns not

22

sour but often bitter. In any case, it tastes bad and can no longer serve as food.

Anyone who still has an unspoiled sense of taste can tell the difference between fresh and pasteurized milk. The difference is still stronger when the milk is heated to about 100°C, which produces the typical 'boiled milk taste.' When the milk is then put straight into airtight containers, so that no bacteria can get in, we have *sterilized milk*. The putrefying bacteria have now also been eliminated. The milk will keep practically forever unless the container is opened.

The 'skin' which forms when milk is heated over 100°C indicates that at least part of the protein has coagulated. Officially this is called 'denaturing' because the protein is no longer natural; it has been changed. Souring also causes coagulation but of a completely different kind. It produces fine, soft, round flocculations that are visible.

As one would expect, the change is even more marked and problematic if the milk is heated to a higher temperature, which can be easily done in closed vessels. It has been known for decades that at temperatures of about 140°C not only the fat changes a great deal, but above all protein changes to such an extent that toxins arise. In spite of this, ultra-heat treatment is more and more widely used today. The milk is brought to a temperature of 135°C to 140°C for about two seconds. This produces *UHT milk* (*u*ltra *h*igh *t*emperature) or *H-milk* (highly heated milk). Bottled under sterile conditions this will keep for weeks without having to be kept cool. This is, of course, extremely practical and therefore misleading to consumers. It is evident that there is no appreciable loss of minerals with this method. Even vitamins may still be found, though at reduced levels. As said before, however, this is not really what matters. It is the level of life which is important. The taste will also have changed in a way that is really impossible to miss, though most people have less sense of taste today and may fail to notice it.

Heating sensitive foods such as milk is therefore a big problem. To object that ultra-heat treatment is 'only' applied for two seconds misses the point. If we were to treat blood in the same way, it would immediately be obvious that it coagulates and can no longer support life. A well-known nutrition expert (Bruker) once compared UHT milk vividly to a corpse that had been stabbed, shot and then hanged. This applies to an even greater degree to *condensed milk*. Milk is thickened by partial evaporation and canned under sterile conditions (in the USA, sugar is also added). This is a massive intervention into the whole structure of the milk, as can be noticed by the complete change in taste when the required amount of water has been added back to the condensed milk. This former milk will undoubtedly also still contain a residue of 'life,' but it has been greatly changed, as the taste shows. It will fill the stomach, and one can even gain weight with it, for it still contains energy—but not life. We will come back to this essential difference.

Sadly, many mothers have no idea what UHT milk really means. In Spanish-speaking countries, for example, it is called *larga vida*, which means 'long life.' Mothers especially buy it to ensure 'long life' for their children. To put it another way, the use of UHT milk will not cause evident damage, but produces a *deficiency* of life that may only become evident after years, or perhaps even generations.

You may say that meat is also exposed to temperatures of 200°C or more when it is fried or roasted and that this does no harm. That is not quite true, as will be seen when meat will be discussed. And compared to milk, meat is extremely 'robust.' Milk is highly sensitive by nature, just like the babies for whom it was created. Babies are distinctly more sensitive and susceptible than adults. This is also why milk changes much more rapidly once it has been 'taken out' of the mother, and changes in a way that differs completely from meat. So it matters a great deal not only *whether* and *what* one does but above all *to whom*.

Measuring calories, minerals, vitamins, etc. serves little purpose when we want to judge quality. But the biological value of food can be determined in *feeding experiments*, though these require more time and effort.

The American physician and scientist F. M. Pottenger did such experiments as early as 1940.[3] Unlike other research scientists who evaluate a nutrition experiment after a few weeks, he did long-term trials, feeding cats with either raw or cooked meat as well as milk treated in four different ways:

1) raw milk
2) pasteurized milk
3) dried milk
4) sweetened condensed milk.

Surprisingly, no differences were seen even when the feeding experiment had run for several weeks. However, Pottenger continued with it over generations of cats. The result, after a period of ten years, was as follows:

Cats fed on raw milk stayed healthy and gave birth normally generation after generation. Cats given heat-treated milk had miscarriages within a few generations, their length of life was reduced, and they developed a number of mostly degenerative diseases as well as malformation of bones, jaws and teeth. The degree of severity depended on the way the milk had been treated. Pasteurized milk caused relatively few changes, while dried milk had distinctly greater negative effects. Condensed milk proved disastrous in view of the above-named general damage; which means it has the least biological value. After about four generations, all animals in that group were sick and no longer able to reproduce. (The taste of condensed milk also differs most from that of fresh milk.) UHT milk was not available at the time. The experiments were repeated with white rats, yielding the same results. Many other research scientists later did similar experiments, practically always with the same result. Kollath, for instance, was but one of them.[4]

The important point in these experiments is that the damaged animals were in no way undernourished, nor did they show the well-known vitamin deficiencies or any toxic symptoms. It was a general weakening in the 'whole' organism, as we call it today: an etheric, life weakness. What really gives pause for thought is that the damage did not show itself immediately but only after one, two or even three generations. Would anyone in our fast-moving day and age consider that the food we eat can have such deep-reaching effects?

Another method of 'processing' milk for the market is *homogenization*. This is done primarily for practical purposes. When milk is left to stand, the cream will rise to the top. After some time the cream clots, and it will not dissolve properly again after this. This thick milk fat is, of course, the best part, the 'crème de la crème.' It is sold as *crème fraiche*, a lightly soured cream with highly concentrated fat. This is why whole milk will go 'lumpy' if left to stand for some time—the fat sticks to the edges of the container, and all one can do is scrape it off. This makes it more difficult to deal with milk in bottles or cartons. Homogenization prevents the cream from clotting. The milk is forced against a surface at high pressure, breaking up the relatively large fat globules into much smaller ones. The main argument in favor of the process is that the milk will then coagulate more evenly in the stomach, making it more digestible. This is true, but the question is why God or nature did not arrange for this in the first place. After all, these two creators have invented things that are much more complicated than this. So why is milk not homogenized by nature? Modern people naturally want to 'improve' nature, but always only for practical or economic reasons. Biological aspects are usually ignored.

When homogenization was introduced, some people pointed out that in normal non-homogenized milk, the bigger, natural globules are not absorbed until they are first emulsified in the intestine to make them digestible. This milk fat is, after all, a foreign fat, and the organism must first destroy it before absorbing it. The fine globules produced by artificial homogenization, however, can now pass directly through the intestinal wall into the bloodstream, where they are not meant to go without being first treated by the intestinal juices. Then, it was aruged, they would be deposited in the blood vessels or cause other problems such as allergies. These arguments were vigorously disputed, but up to today no conclusive experimental work has been done either proving or refuting these views.

Lactic Acid Fermentation

Let us go back to the further fate of milk products. As already mentioned, fresh milk left to itself will turn sour after a time because the ever-present lactobacilli in the air convert the sugar in the milk into lactic acid. In modern cowsheds, the milk has to be cooled down immediately to 5°C to prevent bacterial growth and make the milk keep better. This is a justifiable compromise to allow for milk distribution. This 'cold shock' alters the sensitive milk so that natural souring will not be quite so spontaneous. The taste will also differ from that of milk 'fresh from the cow.'

Certainly lactic acid fermentation is a breaking-down process, and the fine floccular coagulation which results does change the milk protein. It would seem, therefore, that it destroys a significant amount of the life in the milk. Yet people never thought so in the past. Sour milk has been thoroughly enjoyed from early times, more recently with added cinnamon and sugar. The lactobacilli will differ from region to region, so that the resulting product varies. For instance, it is the milk-souring bacteria of Bulgaria that sour our sour milk today, producing what we call 'yogurt.' This is why the bacteria needed for it are called *lactobacillus bulgaricus*. Much more yogurt with Bulgarian souring bacteria is now consumed in central Europe than sour milk with local bacteria, though it was quite unknown there before the First World War. Swedish milk and longmilk (*filmjölk*), both of Scandanavia, are also produced industrially in dairies today using selectively bred lactobacilli. Anyway, the change from milk sugar to lactic acid and the change in protein due to the mild souring certainly do not mean a loss of vitality, in spite of these being breaking-down processes. It is rather a form of predigestion, because milk is also soured in the stomach, which makes it coagulate.

This not only makes it more digestible but also denatures it, which is a first step in coming to grips with the surrounding world and overcoming foreign influences (see 'Understanding Digestive Functions, page 51).

Lactic acid fermentation can happen naturally not only with milk but also with vegetables, especially cucumbers and cabbage. Sour cucumbers and sauerkraut have been produced by this method for centuries all over the world. They were known to have health-giving qualities. To produce them, one does have to use salt to extract the juice from the vegetable, and exclude air to some degree. That is why cucumbers that are prepared like this are called 'salt cucumbers' in German (*Salzgurken*), in contrast to gherkins or 'vinegar cucumbers' (*Essiggurken*) which are the common pickles known worldwide today. Every farmer's wife used to know the natural lactic acid fermentation method in the past. But cucumbers pickled in vinegar have largely taken over as they are easier to produce and keep practically forever. Other vegetables and even fish (Norwegian *gravadlax*) or meat can all be preserved by the lactic acid process. In Russia, *kvass* is still a universally popular drink; it is made from sourdough rye bread. A version of this is sold in central Europe as *Brottrunk* (bread drink). In agriculture, silage is produced in the same way. The acid prevents the growth of putrefying bacteria, which cause rotting. This process will make food keep for some time, though not without limit. The lactic acid also has a general strengthening effect and makes food more digestible. Most people who do not tolerate cabbage or cucumbers have no problem eating sauerkraut or salt cucumbers.

Lactic acid is a kind of 'turntable' in human metabolism where many different metabolic substances meet to initiate new anabolism (constructive metabolism). When a person moves, for instance, the sugar in the muscles of the body is degraded to lactic acid; this lactic acid is then built up again into sugar (glycogen) in the liver. This means that for new synthesis to take place (in the liver) there must first be breakdown (in the muscle)! This relationship is typical of higher life forms where there has to be an *active breaking down process,* which is very different from what happens in plants. But the degree of catabolism (destructive metabolism) of sugar in muscle is actually only a *mild* breaking down process, only going as far as lactic acid and not so far as to become 'waste' (carbon dioxide and water) that has to be eliminated. The liver is able to synthesize most of the lactic acid back into sugar again, with only a small amount of lactic acid being completely 'burned up' for this purpose, that is, broken down into carbon dioxide and water. Lactic acid holds a position between breaking down and building up, between catabolism and anabolism, the two polar-opposite metabolic processes. It enables and indeed guides the transition from breaking down to building up. This is the principle of the middle, and it is healing in character.

This is also what makes it different from *alcoholic* fermentation. *Alcohol* is the end-product of degradation of sugar by yeast. Although it comes from life, unlike lactic acid it cannot be built up again by the body. Alcohol hangs onto the dying process that is in it. This is why it has a conserving and antiseptic action. It also explains why alcohol is a strong poison for the liver, because the liver needs live substances to build up its own live substances again. That is also why most people who have cirrhosis have a long history of excessive alcohol consumption. Alcohol cannot be re-synthesized in the body. It does not stimulate constructive metabolism like lactic acid, but *has* to be burned up completely. (This is why drinks with high alcohol concentrations have a warming effect.) In nature, alcohol can be broken down to acetic acid (i.e., vinegar). Vinegar does not present the acute danger of alcohol, but it also does not contain the nourishing, anabolic, constructive quality of lactic acid. This is why a salad dressing with sour cream and lemon juice, instead of oil and vinegar, is a better contribution to a healthy diet.

However, the real significance of alcohol for human beings is that it hinders the specifically human abilities— the abilities that make humans different from animals. These specifically human capacities are: upright walking, speaking and thinking. That is the sequence in which a child slowly distinguishes itself from animals in the course of development. In alcoholic intoxication, these typically human capacities are affected in reverse order. First the intoxicated person cannot think clearly, then he speaks thickly, then he staggers, until he finally has to crawl on all fours. The disinhibition after intake of even relatively small quantities of alcohol comes from the cutting off of the power of judgment, which belongs to thinking, so that the lower animal instincts show themselves uncontrolled.

In earlier times the lactic acid fermentation process was known all over the world. This 'invention' was surely not based on accidental observation, or because perhaps people did not have refrigerators! Like all old traditions it arose out of profound insight into the influence which food has on human beings. Today, although still used widely, lactic acid fermentation is often not appreciated enough. Still quite familiar is the mentioned Norwegian preservation of salmon by lactic acid fermentation, as well as the Russian custom of the fermentative acidification of cabbage, onions, turnips, and so forth. Certainly a significant aspect of the healthy nutrition in the Ukraine is due to the many different sour milk products consumed there. This procedure was already used in ancient Egypt. Miso in Japan is based on lactic acid fermentation of the soybean. Less familiar is the easily digestible lactic acid fermented chicken of Argentina (*pollo al barro*). In lactic acid fermentation, a process is permitted to occur that could not be achieved by the mere addition of acid.

The way we use milk today is totally contrary to the way it was used in former times. In 'civilized' countries, unsoured milk is produced and consumed in vast quantities. It is often specially recommended for elderly people, with the idea that the calcium contained in milk will slow down or prevent osteoporosis. As in other areas, not only nutrition, overdoing things creates a new problem. It is a fact that an increasing number of children, and also adults, are showing allergic reactions to milk. This undoubtedly has many causes, but this defense reaction against foreign substances, which is the basis of allergies,[6] may also be connected with the reduction of milk quality due to processing methods (see UHT-milk, homogenization, and so forth) and with drinking it at the wrong age. The right age is mainly during childhood, though adults too can drink up to 750 ml of milk daily without ill effect.

Continuing with the processing of milk, the liquid whey will be separated from coagulated sour milk protein. Then we get *quark*, a soft white *curd cheese* which still contains the milk protein and fat. Quark is not just much more digestible than milk, but because it is soured it is the most easily digestible protein of all. It may thus form an important foundation in nutrition.

If the curd is left to stand for a while, specific protein-digesting bacteria will grow on it. A new product comes into being: *cheese.* Starting with the curd and the bacteria that will naturally grow on it, we get a degree of decay which after a period of time gives the typical powerful smell of all matured cheeses.

Again it will depend on the kind of bacteria and the right nutrient base for them. Variation may be produced by heating the milk to a greater or lesser degree before coagulating it. Coagulation can also be effected using an enzyme which breaks down protein. In the past this enzyme (rennet) was obtained from the stomachs of calves, but today it is produced using genetic engineering. Depending on regional variations, different bacteria are involved, and this gives rise to local differences in cheeses, which need months to mature. Cheeses are therefore named according to their place of origin (Cheddar, Edam, Gouda, and so on). These include yellow and hard cheeses (Parmesan, and so on).

The manufacturing processes and the specific bacteria needed are known today, so that Edam cheese, for instance, can be produced all over the world, though the flavor is often very different from the original—so much so that it does not take an expert to be aware of it.

Inoculation with specific molds will take the process further, producing strong-tasting 'delicacy cheeses' such as gorgonzola, roquefort, blue cheese, camembert and others. The process of breaking down the protein may also go so far that putrefying substances develop out of decaying protein. This one can smell. Also substances such as tyramine are produced which can trigger headaches or migraine in susceptible individuals. Those who have this sensitivity should avoid all cheeses which are too ripe and therefore strongly 'perfumed' and aromatic (ripe strong-smelling yellow and hard cheeses and all mold cheeses), but may consume curd (quark). They must also avoid chocolate, which also contains such substances. In particular, large quanities of mold cheese may also affect the intestinal flora. There can be no objection to eating such 'delicacies' by people who are not sensitive to them, provided they are eaten in the small amounts appropriate for delicacies.

Vitality and Fertility

The role of nutrition in health has recently become a topic from quite a different angle. The number of couples unable to have children for biological reasons is known to be increasing. For a long time this was thought to be the woman's problem, for that used to be the way of thinking. However, a number of recently published papers have shown that sperm quality has been deteriorating dramatically over the last 70 years. The men affected are not really sick; they 'simply' lack vitality (*not* sexuality).

Investigations published in recent years have provided clear evidence that *fertility* is largely dependent on nutrition. More than 60 years ago it was found that the fertility of breeding bulls was decreasing in spite (or because?) of the concentrates they were fed. It was restored by feeding hay from unfertilized high alpine meadows. Experimental work later confirmed these findings and added to them. Comparison was made between rabbits given fodder produced in the conventional way and others given biodynamically produced fodder (Demeter quality). It is important to note that there was no difference in the composition of the fodder as far as the nutrients were concerned, nor in the usual analyses, vitamin content for instance. In spite of this, the biodynamically produced fodder gave the rabbits better health and fertility. Thus the pregnancy rate was the same for both groups in the first generation. In the second generation it was 59% with conventional fodder and 86% with biodynamic fodder. Similar distinct differences were seen in the number of live births per litter. Susceptibility to infection also showed marked differences in the second generation. Other investigations showed the same results: organic or biodynamic fodder improves fertility and health, whereas intensive use of mineral fertilizer has a negative effect.[7]

How is it possible to have such different effects? The reason is that we do not know what life really is, where it comes from, and how it is connected with physical substances. But we can know today that life is a force. It is transformed light, as we have discussed earlier. And only certain substances—foods, the 'mediators of life'—contain life, or ought to contain it.

Although the above-mentioned investigations were done a long time ago (see chapters on milk, pages 22f), hardly any notice was taken of them. And the conclusions were not put into practice. We can definitely conclude that the effect of food goes deep, impacting the life of the whole organism. This starts with the methods of cultivating the plants, which play an essential role. Processing also has a major influence. Preservation of any kind will not retain the life in food over the long term. Suitable methods can however make the most out of the life forces, for instance lactic fermentation of milk.

Nevertheless, compromises will have to be accepted today. The above investigations were cited in detail to enable readers to judge how far we should go with such compromises.

The Role of Vitamins

The crucial question to what extent a food actually still contains life, which can only come from a living substance, is also important in another area. The freshly pressed juice of a healthy fruit or vegetable clearly still contains life forces that can nourish people. It has been shown that these can only be *partially* preserved. But human beings always want to 'improve' on nature, so the 'unnecessary parts' of a juice or vegetable are removed from those that are wanted. When nutrition first began as a science, it was declared that only the 'energy content' and usable substances mattered. Thus, the indigestible parts of grains or rice were removed, and people were proud to have snowy white flour or rice. This went well in fact for some time in the case of rice. Then people began to develop strange symptoms such as paralysis and other forms of nerve damage. The condition was given the name 'beriberi.' Later it was found that people were missing something. And the missing 'something' was found in the very hulls which had been thrown out or fed to the pigs.

So began the search for the missing substance, and a substance was actually found! Chemically it proved to be an amine (the smallest fragment of protein). It clearly was a carrier of life (Latin *vita*). And so the term 'vitamin' was created, to refer to the very essence of any substance which human beings cannot produce themselves and therefore must take in with their food to remain healthy. This first vitamin was vitamin B (from 'beriberi'). Later, others were found and named using letters of the alphabet. By definition, vitamins are thus substances which the organism is not able to produce itself. They have to be supplied from outside. Requirements differ in different species. Most animals are able to produce their own vitamin C, which therefore is not a vitamin in their case. Humans—and strangely enough, guinea pigs—are unable to do so. They must take in vitamin C with their food. It is found in all fresh fruit and vegetables. If vitamin C, or rather fresh food, is lacking, people develop scurvy. It used to be common among seafarers on long journeys where no fresh food was available. Symptoms were hemorrhaging, extreme weakness, and loosening and falling out of teeth,

Vitamins do indeed come from a living process. For a long time they were therefore thought to be the essence of health. Unfortunately, it was discovered too late that over-dosage can cause severe damage. This was noted particularly with vitamin D. We know now that vitamin D is not actually a vitamin but rather a hormone which the body is able to produce itself. Provitamin D, the hormone produced by the body, is able to take up light, which activates it. In this case, the real vitamin which has to come from outside is therefore light. The substance itself, provitamin D, only acts as a mediator. Childhood rickets can therefore be prevented or cured with either light or vitamin D. Vitamin D is 'sunlight captured in a test tube,' as one pediatrician has put it (von Pfaundler).

Through light irradiation it was now easy to produce artificial vitamin D and administer it in high doses. Rickets (the 'English disease'), a condition in which not enough calcium is deposited in the bones, disappeared completely through the use of vitamin D. However, the opposite then happened: premature calcification, causing severe sclerosis and sometimes even death. It took years before it was realized that this was due to vitamin D over-dosage.

Cod liver oil has a particularly high vitamin D content. However, this will not be harmful because the high fat content prevents excessive intake (by causing diarrhea). In addition, cod liver oil (like butter) also contains vitamin A, which counteracts vitamin D (so long as the oil is not technically processed and the two vitamins are *naturally* bound together). While vitamin D causes deposits, hardening and calcification, vitamin

A is involved in metabolic processes that dissolve and build up. This is why vitamin A and vitamin E, which is similar to it, are often recommended to prevent hardening, for instance in the heart (heart attack). Vitamins A, D and E are fat-soluble, vitamins B and C water-soluble. Having a one-sided view of vitamins as being essential to life, people believe that the whole health issue is now completely 'under control' with vitamins. Thus, vitamin D is added to all milk in the USA in the belief that the human organism 'needs' it to strengthen the bones. Older women in particular are advised to consume lots of milk (and milk products) to which extra vitamin D has been added in order to 'prevent' possible osteoporosis. Vitamin D essentially 'forces' the organism to take up calcium, but it does not determine where it is to be deposited. The calcium in blood may then be deposited in irregularities in the vascular walls instead of being deposited in the bones. This may lead to the grotesque situation that blood vessels calcify more than the bones do. If calcium deposits form in the vessels that supply the heart or the brain, conditions may arise that ultimately lead to heart attack or poor cerebral blood circulation (even to the point of causing dementia).[1]

Bone grows brittle with osteoporosis because there is a loss of elasticity. But elasticity depends on silica, not calcium. Calcium makes bones hard, and precisely because of this it also makes them brittle. (The same phenomenon is also seen in glass, for instance, which is hard and therefore breaks easily.) Contrary to calcium, organic silica binds great quantities of water to itself, creating a substance that is half solid and half fluid, that is, elastic. Organs rich in silica and therefore elastic are cartilage, skin, hair, nails and connective tissue in general. Rye, millet, barley and horsetail (equisetum) have a high silica content. Also gelatin bought in health food stores, or produced by boiling animal bones to dissolve the cartilage in them, is rich in silica. These should be eaten in quantity (e.g. gelatin in soup) in cases of osteoporosis. Cartilage is found not only on the surfaces of the joints but is also responsible for the elasticity of all long bones, whose matrix is made of cartilage. In osteoporosis, cartilage levels in the bones are reduced (just as they are in osteoarthritis) and as a result the bones are no longer elastic, but brittle.

Further investigations led to the identification of many vitamin subgroups (B1, B6, B12) as well as further vitamins, for instance, vitamin F in fats, later identified as unsaturated fatty acids (see page 96). Finally it became evident that the term 'vitamin' does not always apply. This is why in recent times, the chemical names of the substances have come to be used instead (vitamin C = ascorbic acid, vitamin B1 = thiamine, and so forth).

Vitamins are indeed highly active substances and the carriers of specific vital processes. These may be stimulated by giving the corresponding vitamins in relatively high doses. But it is not so much the isolated substances which matter, it is the substances in their relationship to the whole context. Meanwhile many people are not taking only the daily recommended dose but megadoses, that is, many times the amount of vitamins present in food. This may occasionally serve a purpose in some diseases, but it does not change the general situation of nutrition. On the contrary, it may lead to situations where the increased dose will no longer be effective and has to be increased further—a vicious circle without end.

Sugar: Energy Source without Life

Since life needs a watery environment, plant saps, milk or blood contain the wholeness of life forces. It is human nature to want to have 'pure' pleasure, with nothing else mixed in. In practice this means when we have a sweet fruit juice, we want it still sweeter. This led people not just to use the juice pressed from the quite sweet sugar cane but to concentrate it, removing any part that was not sweet. This produced the essence of sweetness, refined white sugar that is 99.97% pure. The concentration and refining processes were soon done on an industrial scale. Factory-made sugar became cheap and available in large quantities. Later, beets were specially bred to produce relatively high concentrations of sugar. This has become the sugar generally used in Europe because sugar cane only grows in hot climates. But refining has reached such a high degree that there is practically no difference now between the two kinds of sugar. This is why it is not possible to taste whether a piece of sugar comes from sugar cane or from sugar beets.

What does this 'purifying' mean? No living creature consists of only one pure substance. The infinite variety of life depends on a wide variety of substances in order to take effect. This immediately tells us that an isolated substance, whatever it may be, cannot be a carrier of life anymore. At best it will have preserved a very small portion of life. Sugar does in fact still have this small portion, but it is no longer life, which depends on variety—it is merely 'energy.' Anyone can notice this: When we have reached the end of our strength after hard physical labor, or perhaps after a strenuous shopping expedition in town, the fatigue can be instantly overcome with sugar, and of course it will even be more effective in a cup of coffee. We feel new 'energy,' and in this context that is the right word! But in a 'sugar high,' we fail to notice that this energy is not life. It is *borrowed* energy, energy taken in directly, without effort. No food can or should enter directly into the bloodstream, except for sugar! Anything else must first be digested and inwardly processed. This is why sugar energy is not something we have gained through our own effort; it is really something we have 'stolen' from nature, literally in a 'refined,' that is, sophisticated way.

It is most important to realize that pure sugar does not exist in nature! The highest concentrations of sugar are found in honey, which is rare and difficult to obtain in its natural setting. Honey is not at all the same as sugar, for it also contains many enzymes and vitamins, all of which are carriers of life. These come from the flowers as well as from the bees. Honey was therefore traditionally used more as a medicine than as a food.

It will be clear by now that such energy, the strength that one gets from sugar, is actually an illusion. One can already see this from the fact that the effect disappears after just a few hours. A reactive drop in blood sugar to subnormal levels follows and is felt as tiredness and hunger. What better solution than to take more sugar again? A 'sugar craving' develops, truly a vicious circle which many people are caught in today. This has been discussed in more detail elsewhere.[8]

One only has to look closely at sugar to understand this. Sugar is a crystal. Crystals are never living. They are typical representatives of the non-living world. Crystals in the mineral world do not, of course, contain 'energy,' which is a special property of sugar. Because sugar has energy, it can be burned. But like all crystals, sugar is a dead substance. In fact, sugar is not just dead, in concentrated form it even can kill. It can be used to make preserves such as home-made or factory-made jam. When the fruit is boiled with at least 50% sugar ('pound for pound,' as housewives say when they make jam) the fruit will not ferment, as yeast cannot live in such sugar concentrations (60% sugar is considered absolutely safe; the product will then keep indefinitely; at 50%, mold or fermentation may still occur).

The essential point is that sugar does not provide life, but only energy. And this is why no human being or animal can live only on sugar, precisely because it does not have life. People are aware of this today; it is known that vitamin B is needed to digest sugar. If there is none available, sugar becomes a vitamin B robber. In the long run this again means damage, above all to the nervous system. In nature, there is built-in prevention. The starch in a kernel of grain or rice transforms very quickly into sugar when eaten. But it is surrounded with vitamin B from the hull, which is needed to digest the sugar. In highly refined flour, however, this hull is removed. In some countries, therefore, the law requires adding vitamin B to white flour— and in accordance with today's way of thinking, it will be the *synthetic* vitamin. Methods do exist for dissolving the natural vitamin out of the hull and introducing it into the starchy part (parboiled rice). It is a question, however, what other effects such industrial processes may produce. It should be clear that only the whole grain still retains the wholeness of life.

From the above discussion, it is evident that it is better and more natural to grind and use the whole grain rather than refine it to produce snowy white flour and then re-intoduce synthetic vitamins, iron and other things that were first removed. This will not result in a product of 'whole grain' value. We cannot produce an organism such as a whole grain by 'putting parts together,' even if adding in the missing part may avoid the worst health problems (see 'The Role of Vitamins,' page 36).

What has been said so far should give a basis for judging what is important in nutrition: what we are actually taking in or may not be getting, namely *life* with its various qualities. Real obstacles exist, however. It is hardly possible for anyone who wants to have completely healthy nutrition today to do so. The products one would need are not always available. It canot be a matter of avoiding every single gram of sugar or the occasional dash of condensed milk or sterilized cream to make a cup of coffee tastier. (Even people with a fine palate no longer notice the difference from fresh cream.) Such situations sometimes call for compromise. However, *long*-term consumption of abundant 'maltreated' milk, sugar or canned food will cause considerable damage or deficiencies—especially in children, who depend more than adults on immediate life in order to grow. The damage is not generally noticed. Nowadays the sugar consumption of children and young people is often unrestrained. And it is well known that the health of today's children, or rather their general vitality (not one or more specific diseases, but the health of their whole constitution) is rapidly decreasing. But people will only rarely see the connection of this fact with nutrition.

Cancer too is greatly influenced by food. It has been shown scientifically that a tumor has a fermenting metabolism, not a putrefying metabolism. That is, cancer cells feed on sugar, not on protein or fat. This fact is even used in some chemotherapies, where a concentrated sugar solution is given to the patient beforehand. This intensifies the metabolism of the cancer cells, so that they absorb more chemo-therapeutic medications. But if one eats sugar *without* the toxic chemotherapy, one feeds the tumor cells directly. Starch, which easily becomes sugar, also has this effect. So a cancer patient should not only avoid all sugar (see page 18) but also starch—that is, potatoes, husked grains (white rice, etc.) and white flour (white bread, noodles).

The Problem of Food Additives

The many *additives* in foods further aggravate the problem. This starts with the agrochemicals (insecticides, pesticides, etc.) used to 'save the crops.' (It is a common refrain: 'All we have left to eat is what the pests leave us.') In reality most 'pests' are indicators of something being not right, for instance use of excessive amounts of fertilizer. Monoculture offers an invitation to other creatures to come and 'help themselves.' On the other hand, selective breeding aiming only at high yields creates a one-sidedness in plants and animals. This calls for correction in the wholeness of nature. So-called pests make the correction, just as so-called weeds tend to balance out deficiencies in the soil. Therefore, in reality they are often the remedy for a maltreated soil. Eco*logy* has luckily developed a great deal in recent times. It involves the study of interconnections and relationships in nature and among living beings. This is in contrast to eco*nomy*, which has so far been dominant, a science where the focus is on profitability.

In most cases, the 'chemical club' is used to combat undesirable insects or plants. Of course residues remain on food, but the real problem is that the whole approach is fundamentally wrong. In the long run, nature will react and hit back. It took decades of DDT use, which was highly effective, before people realized that the insects were growing resistant. The outstanding weapon had thus become completely ineffective. Nevertheless, DDT has spread all over the world and is now present in the fat of practically all mammals and human beings. The battle against malaria, so promising at first, has in effect also been lost. The relatively harmless forms of malaria (*tertiary*) have practically vanished. Instead highly aggressive forms have gained the upper hand (*plasmodium falciparum* and *vivax*). We have the same situation with bacteria which are growing resistant to antibiotics.

Only small amounts of insecticides, pesticides and other 'plant protectives' actually get into the food. However, untold numbers of 'improvers' are added during processing, from preservatives to coloring agents, emulsifiers, stabilizers, thickeners, flavors, flavor enhancers, and many more additives for which no declaration is needed. In the USA, for instance, around 2700 food additives are permitted that do not have to be declared at all. They have, of course, all been 'tested,' though it is not clear how and for how long those tests were conducted.

As German humorist Wilhelm Busch (1832-1908) once pointed out, human nature is 'cunning and clever,' always trying to make things better. Therefore we have been trying for a long time to imitate and, of course, improve on nature. But this is only apparently possible. It is true that a good meal should not be only nourishing and healthy but also tasty. Flavor and aroma are real quality criteria. The art of cooking lies in maintaining these or even helping them to unfold. Heat has been used for this purpose from the earliest days. Generally speaking, the higher the temperature, the more intense the aroma and taste. When meat is cooked, for instance, it develops a special aroma that is stronger than that of raw meat. The aroma gets that much more intense, however, when it is fried. Coffee beans develop their aroma only through roasting, which uses even higher tempera- tures than frying. Humanity has made an art of all these methods. They also serve to ripen the food to some extent, but they always require time. Nowadays people do not have time, and this is why many aromas have been artificially produced. They are manufactured today by the ton, and technically this is no longer a problem. A single factory will produce about 7,000 different aromatic components, from pineapple to lemon flavor. If declared at all, the label usually just says 'nature-identical aromas.' That is misleading, to say the least. Every natural aroma or scent is made up of not one but a large number of substances that serve as carriers. Synthetic production usually only means a single substance for strawberry or banana flavor.

But this one substance offers a tremendous advantage: the aroma can be added in practically any amount. A product that may otherwise be rather tasteless will then have a powerful flavor. The one-sidedness will be tasted immediately, for instance with synthetic ('nature-identical') strawberry flavor. Natural vanilla flavor has been found to contain about forty different substances. Synthetic vanillin is a single, chemically 'pure' substance. Its flavor is not only stronger, of course, but also quite one-sided. It is actually 'kitsch'—artificial instead of the truly 'artistic' aroma created by nature. Now, human taste buds have got so used to the strength and one-sidedness of synthetic vanillin that the majority of consumers recognize the taste of vanillin as the 'real' vanilla taste. They ask for synthetic vanillin. The subtler natural aroma seems tasteless to most people today. Vanillin is therefore used in almost every vanilla ice cream and in practically every chocolate. Modern consumers have been exposed to the excessive sensory stimulus of synthetic vanillin since childhood and are used to it. It is also a question of the availability of the natural substance in such large quantities. If natural vanilla pods were to be used to flavor the vast amounts of vanilla ice cream and chocolate consumed all over the world, almost the entire tropics would need to be covered with this plant.

The way human taste sensations are being fixed on one substance as the characteristic taste, a taste that is in fact one-sided and 'off the mark,' is a corruption of human sense organs that goes unnoticed. It is an expression of the general flooding of the senses with stimuli and information, whose rising amounts can no longer be controlled. As a result, over-stimulation leads to a general dulling of the senses. Weaker, subtler stimuli can no longer be felt. Quantity prevails over quality, and people's general scale of values becomes one-sided and coarse.

In this way it is possible, for instance, to produce 'chicken soup' without any chicken or 'vanilla ice cream'without (real) vanilla, and so on. By starting with a basic product which is intentionally kept neutral and easy to package, the addition of aroma + color + generous amounts of salt or sugar can transform it into the perfect and even cheap illusion. Infinite such possibilities have opened up and are eagerly put to use.

In spite of the problems of the synthetically produced 'nature-identical' substances we have been discussing, it must be said that they are a bit closer to the human metabolism than the many *purely* synthetic products which have never existed before.* These may be highly effective, but they make demands on the body for which it has not been designed.

Flavor enhancers act in a different way. Many of them exist in nature. First and foremost among them is salt. A dish that is one hundred percent salt free has almost no taste at all! Higher animals, especially goats, love salt. Humans are the greatest salt lovers; they are practically addicted to it. In earlier times, when transport facilities were not yet what they are today, salt was literally worth its weight in gold. Well-salted dishes have a more intense taste, which does not mean they taste better. Ordinary table salt (sodium chloride) is essential for the function of nerves. For plants it is poison, with just a few exceptions. We can already see from this that salt belongs to humans and animals. Its significance lies not principally in the sphere of biological processes but more in higher functions, in consciousness. It is rather a mediator of

---

* The word 'nature-identical' means that this substance has been chemically synthesized, but is chemically the same as a substance which exists in plants or animals. Contrary to 'artifical aromas' which chemically do not exist in nature, the 'nature-identical aromas' are allowed to be put in food without any previous testing.

pleasure, a sort of stimulant. This was known 2000 years ago. The Latin word *sal* means not only 'salt' but also 'wit,' in the sense of heightened consciousness. Eating a lot of salt not only raises the blood pressure, but as a result also makes reactions faster. The individual is more 'wide awake,' and this is considered desirable. However, a constantly raised blood pressure may lead to a number of diseases.

Some years ago the specific flavor-enhancing effect of monosodium glutamate was discovered. This is an amino acid derived from protein. It is widely used, especially in Chinese cookery. Excessive use has a powerful temporary stimulant effect, followed by an equally powerful tiredness. Smaller amounts of monosodium glutamate are still added to food today, above all to ready meals.

Sugar is also a strong flavor enhancer. This is why it is often added to salty foods (tomato ketchup contains about 14% sugar!). Nowadays not only every brand of cucumber pickled in vinegar, but also fish preserves and fish salad have sugar or synthetic sweetener added to intensify and 'round out' the flavor.

It should be obvious from the above that such constant, one-sided 'stimulation' will gradually blunt the sense of taste. The unadulterated product will not seem very attractive anymore, and subtleties of taste tend to be lost. In reality this constant over-stimulation represents an impoverishment! The same applies to the other senses. Constant background music and continually changing lights in garish colors overwhelm the senses and our ability to listen carefully and reflect. Ultimately our inner life is impoverished.

Most of the additives mentioned serve to make products appear better than they really are by adding color, aroma and so on. To put it bluntly, this is fraud, since something is suggested that is not present. The number of additives is so vast that it is impossible to keep track of them, let alone of the interactions between them and their long-term effects.

It has been known for a long time that many of these substances may trigger allergies, but the number of additives is so vast that it is hardly possible to determine which is the substance that produces the allergy.

In 1965, Benjamin Feingold,[9] a California pediatrician and allergy expert, found that a patient lost her physical allergic reactions once she excluded all synthetic food additives from her diet. Her psychic symptoms, which had persisted for two years, also improved markedly.

Over the next ten years he saw similar responses in others, especially in the many cases of hyperactive boys. The boys were evidently showing hypersensitive reactions to specific food additives. Feingold went on to develop a 'diet,' the 'only' rule being that all synthetic additives must be completely avoided. Many of the parents who took his advice saw their children's behavior improve in just a few weeks. However, the improvement would disappear as soon as the children went back to eating food containing synthetic additives. Here again it is also important to avoid all sugar for at least four weeks (see page 18).

At almost the same time pharmacist Hertha Hafer[10] noted that sedatives seriously aggravated the condition of her hyperactive child who had severe behavioral problems. Stimulants brought transient improvement. She finally discovered that a particular class of additives that does not have to be declared would trigger the symptoms. These are the phosphates added to soft drinks, instant dissolving beverages (such as instant cocoa powder), all sausages, cheese spreads, etc. Phosphates do not have to be declared because they are natural substances. But what is *not* natural is the *quantity* of phosphate that is added to these products. Complete avoidance of these foods and sugar improves the children's condition in a remarkably short time (four weeks). Many parents can confirm this, but Hafer's findings, as well as those of Feingold, have been officially rejected. Parents have therefore formed self-help groups in many areas (Phosphate League).[11]

Why is it that these very small amounts of additives can trigger both physical (allergy) and psychological (hyperactivity) intolerance reactions in some people, and especially in children? Human beings depend on the natural world. They live on it. Yet nature must not enter into the human organism without being changed first (see 'Understanding Digestive Functions,' page 51). Most of these additives are foreign substances which do not exist in nature, and the human metabolism is not designed for them. Natural processes to protect the biological self from foreign life develop in the course of life. Children must first acquire their immune defenses, but these defense processes do not respond to synthetic substances. Thus the additives are able to enter into the organism 'uninvited' and are only recognized as foreign substances afterwards, when it is too late. The consequence is allergic reactions, though in this case it is not true allergy but hypersensitivity. It may also happen that the organism shows no defensive reactions at all. Its vital processes can be blocked or undergo pathological changes, as they would under a poison. The organism itself is thus switched off and can no longer control itself.

Some of these additives already existed a hundred years ago. It is evident, however, that the use of additives has increased by leaps and bounds in recent years. It seems that the limit of tolerance has been reached, at least in a growing number of people. What is so grotesque about it all is that most additives are put in to improve appearance, and are therefore entirely superfluous from the point of view of nutrition. However, it will take a change in consumer habits and demands to change this increasing risk to people's health.

Understanding Digestive Functions

As mentioned above, the purpose of nutrition is to provide human beings with life. Life differs greatly, however, in the different carriers of life. The starch in potato differs from that in a grain of wheat. In the same way cat protein differs from beef protein, and so on. Cats have presumably been eating mice for millennia, and mice have a different kind of body protein than cats. What would happen if mouse protein got into the cat's blood unchanged? It would mean that in the course of time the cat would become all mouse protein. Inevitably this would change not only the fur, but the whole form and also the animal's behavior. In other words, the cat would gradually turn into a mouse. To prevent this from happening, higher organisms have a digestive system. Its function is to break down foreign life and prevent it from getting in as it is. In other words, the digestive system protects the self from non-self—from foreign life which would make one's own organism into something alien.

Although life is extremely varied and all-encompassing, only three basic substances are found in our food. These are proteins, fats and carbohydrates. It is highly significant that no living organism contains just one of the three on its own. They must always work together to provide a basis for life. Accordingly, there are also three different kinds of digestion.

Protein

Protein is the main body substance of humans and animals. It is not found only in egg (as implied by the German *Eiweiss*, which means both egg white and protein). Muscle, internal organs, skin, and so on also consist largely of it. Protein calls for the most intensive digestion. This begins in the stomach, where the mucous lining produces specific juices for this purpose. These include a powerful acid (hydrochloric acid) and an enzyme called pepsin, which together 'denature' the protein, causing it to coagulate. It is then no longer bound up so intensively with its original life. This also makes it more accessible to further processing in other parts of the gastrointestinal tract. The juices produced by the pancreas break down the substance further. Digestive juices from the small intestine then reduce the protein to amino acids, commonly known as the 'building blocks' of protein. The purpose of the whole process, which is actually one of destruction, is that the specific nature of the protein is removed. It is now no longer chicken or beef protein. It is not foreign anymore, but 'neutral.' It is only now that the very fine fragments can be taken up through the intestinal wall. They pass through the portal vein into the liver.

This digestive process is undoubtedly one of catabolism or destruction. One might think that all the life is now gone, and all that remains of the living protein would be a more or less dead amino acid. This is only partly the case. As the 'destruction' occurs *inside* the organism, the forces of life liberated in the process can stimulate the organism's own life body (ether body). For life, like light, is a force that is only bound up with physical substance for limited periods of time. Now life is freed inside the organism.

Resynthesis in the liver follows, producing specific cat, bovine or human protein, as the case may be. In the process, the forces of life are bound again to substance. The amino acids are not completely dead either. They are processed further in the internal metabolism, being either re-synthesized or broken down into highly active substances of hormone character that are essential for life. Adrenalin is an example.

Problems may arise at different stages of protein degra-dation. If degradation is insufficient, or so much protein is eaten that the organism cannot process it all, the undigested protein reaches the large intestine, where it is broken down by bacteria. This process differs from the breaking down in the small intestine in that it is now one of putrefaction, a rotting process as in nature outside the body. Some of the substances produced are highly toxic. Being soluble they are taken back up into the body and need to be detoxified in the liver. This in turn puts a strain on the liver.

The hydrochloric acid and the pepsin produced in the stomach serve not only to make the protein 'digestible' in the first place, but can also simply digest any undesirable foreign life, such as bacteria, which are also composed of protein. Experiments done with volunteers have shown that cholera bacilli, for instance, do not infect individuals if there is enough hydrochloric acid in their stomach. If the acid is diluted, the bacteria survive passage through the stomach and can later spread in the intestine and cause cholera to develop. Unfortunately the modern habit of drinking before or during the meals dilutes the gastric acid, which favors infection, especially in warmer climates or in conditions where cleanliness is not adequate. *Sweet* drinks (as well as desserts) increase the risk because the composition of saliva and digestive juices changes depending on whether it is sweetness or meat we taste or smell. On the other hand, adding lemon juice to a dish or a salad will help to protect against bacteria.[12]

If protein has been predigested in the stomach but is not yet completely broken down, it is small enough to pass through the intestinal wall. However, since it still has foreign characteristics, the body reacts and tries to eliminate this 'semi-protein' through the skin. This causes skin eruptions. It is one way in which food allergy shows itself.

Omitting these foods will help, of course, but this is not enough. Instead, we must stimulate the digestive functions. This may be done with sour food or bitters (bitter tea as an aperitif), but not with sweet drinks. People have also always known that hot spices, especially mustard and horseradish, will help with the digestion of meat.

Fats

Fats demand less of the digestion. Fat globules, which are relatively large, must first be reduced in size to be taken up into the body. This is the function of bile, a fluid produced by the liver. It emulsifies the fats, making the fat globules small enough to be combined with water. The fats in milk, cream and mayonnaise are already emulsified and therefore more easily digested than solid fats like butter. Later, in the digestive tract, the fat is broken down into fatty acids and glycerin, which can then be taken up into the body.

Bile production and with it the ability to digest fats also depends on the time of the day. The greatest volume of bile is available in the morning and during the day. The process is at rest during the night. Therefore anything fried eaten in the evening—possibly with french fries and mayonnaise!—is a challenge for the gall bladder, which is now empty. The body will frantically try to squeeze the last drops of bile from the gall bladder, which causes an attack of biliary dyspepsia. So this is a problem connected with life rhythms. Eaten at midday, the same meal would usually provoke no such reaction. The classic English breakfast of ham and eggs respects this rhythm, stimulating bile excretion in the morning and therefore also stimulating the individual's activity. For bile makes the human being active. Activity in its turn encourages the flow of bile, even to the point of 'explosion,' as may be seen in cholerics. They are 'bile people' (from the Greek *chole* for 'bile'). If they cannot discharge their activity to the outside it will turn inwards: they turn 'green and blue' with rage, as the German saying goes. In this case, the bile does not go into the intestine but backwards into the blood and the skin, and this is dangerous; they poison themselves. Eggs, fats, fried food and roasted products such as coffee will stimulate bile production the most. People with gall bladder problems should therefore avoid them, especially in the evening.

Carbohydrates

Carbohydrates are even easier to digest. As an experiment, if you chew a piece of bread or boiled potato for a few minutes, you will notice a sweet taste developing. This is because saliva contains an enzyme by which the starch in the bread is reduced already in the mouth to glucose. It is an amazing fact that practically all vegetables and plants are based on this one substance: glucose. Glucose is condensed into starch and stored by plants, as in grains or potatoes. It can be broken down into sugar again as in fruits. Finally, as the plant ages, the starch may condense further to form indigestible cellulose. The woodiness of old vegetables is evidence of this.

This type of digestion also calls for some activity. If there is no activity, or people eat too much sugar, the sugar will reach the large intestine where, just as we saw with protein, microorganisms will 'go on a feeding frenzy.' In the case of protein, these were the putrefactive bacteria, but here it is the yeasts which are 'happy,' as they live on sugar. Yeasts ferment sugar into alcohol—grape juice into wine or malt into beer, for example. It is also yeast that makes bread rise by releasing carbon dioxide. Of course, these intestinal yeasts are not the same as those used in beer brewing and by bakers. They are not cultivated but 'wild' forms. However this may be, their metabolism differs from the metabolism inside the human body where sugar is mainly reduced to lactic acid, as shown earlier. In the process of alcoholic fermentation, wild yeasts produce not only 'pure' alcohol like cultivated yeast, but also many intermediate products the equivalent of 'rotgut.' These substances are very soluble so that they are easily absorbed and may seriously upset the human metabolism. Headaches, tiredness, bad moods and a vast number of different problems may arise as a result.

The fact is that sugar consumption has risen enormously in the 'civilized' world in recent decades. The average per capita intake of sugar in the U.S. is 140 grams (5 oz.) a day—sugar consumption exceeds flour consumption there. The human organism is continually flooded with more sugar than it is able to cope with. Yet sugar requires practically no effort at all for its digestion. This means that we do not develop the capacity *ourselves* to produce the sugar we need from the starch in bread or vegetables. This leads to a general weakening of digestive activity. As a result the organism is progressively less able to control the sugar. This explains why it becomes good soil for the microorganisms which live on sugar outside the organism, namely yeasts. Like all microorganisms, yeasts are highly adaptable and changeable. No wonder that yeasts, which are only fungi and are harmless in themselves, will now colonize not only the whole intestine but also other organs like the lung, and may even cause fatal damage. It ought to be clear that the fault lies not in these 'bad' yeasts but in faulty behavior on the part of humans. People are then no longer 'master in their own house.'

Essentially, the situation is the same as that described for protein. Overloading the organism with protein leads to putrefaction, while too much sugar results in alcoholic fermentation, in either case a kind of process that should not take place *inside* the organism.

It was mentioned above that in the inner metabolism of the human organism sugar is reduced to lactic acid. Lactic acid is also produced outside the human organism in sour milk, lactic acid fermentation of cucumbers, sauerkraut (fermented cabbage)—and in bread baking with sourdough. This involves a problem which has so far been ignored. We will consider it in detail in the chapter on bread baking (page 66).

To sum up, one may say that the purpose of digestion is not only to provide life but also to *make an effort* in order to obtain this life. In digestion, we have to come to grips with physical substance in a most intimate way and change it. The strength to do so has to be developed in childhood; babies only have this capacity as a *possibility*. Such development also enhances the capacity to resist what is 'foreign,' as has been shown. When defense of the self from the non-self takes place inside the body, it is called an 'immune response.' This too, has to be developed in the course of time. Digestion is a first way of practicing it and is an important part of the immune system. This immune system needs to be *developed*. It will be weak unless it is exercised. Rudolf Steiner put the relationship between eating and digestion very succinctly: 'Man eats himself sick and digests himself healthy.'

Bread

The baking of grain into bread undoubtedly goes back to times when the whole of life was still a deeply religious experience. A last vestige of this is seen is the central role which bread continues to play in religious rites. This way of processing grain must have come from ancient mystery knowledge. After all, the principal Christian prayer still says, 'Give us this day our daily bread.'

To bake bread, grain must first be ground. In earlier times this was done slowly between two stones. Already in this method there has been a great deal of change today, for metals are now widely used instead of stones in milling technology. It has been found that temperatures may go up as high as 1000°C at certain points in the milling metals. Clearly this means that the sensitive protein in the grain is changed, if nothing else. Traces of metal from the machinery may also cause aging in the active principles that are liberated in the milling process.

Many different varieties of grain were grown in the past. They were originally bred from grasses a very long time ago. Many of them are today no longer economical to breed. Thus 95% of the many varieties of wheat that used to be grown have died out over the last 100 years. The same holds true for rice. Around the year 1900, 50,000 varieties of rice were grown in India. Today, 10% of them make up 90% of all rice grown. In recent years, however, researchers have started work to save older varieties.

Only a very few generations ago, rye was the main bread grain among Europeans, while wheat was used for pastries and cakes. This has changed dramatically in recent decades. Today, *wheat* is generally considered to be *the* bread grain. There is a problem here that is not recognized. Mice fed entirely on wheat and prevented from eating anything else were found to die after a time, for wheat protein is of limited quality; thus, it lacks one amino acid, lysine, which is essential for life. The varied diet we eat today does, of course, make up for this deficit, but we cannot deny that it exists in wheat. This is also true of whole wheat and whole wheat bread. Rye definitely has more nutritional value. This is why in earlier times bread used to be made out of rye in Europe. Rye bread, not wheat bread, was also given to soldiers. This should make us think. Soldiers need to be healthy and strong, which can be achieved through rye rather than through wheat. Similarly prisoners, who had nothing but bread and water to eat, were given sourdough rye bread and mostly remained healthy in spite of heavy physical labor.

This issue also has a geographical aspect. Wheat grows in warmer regions, rye in cooler climates. The truth is that the things that grow in different climates are 'right' for the living beings in those regions. The Eskimos have a very different diet in their natural habitat than people living in the tropics. If their diets were switched, *both* would become sick! Of course, this refers to the staple food and does not mean that one 'should not' use lemons in cold climates because they do not grow there. The problem is the one-sidedness: wheat has replaced practically all other grains throughout the world.

In 1893, for instance, the ratio of rye to wheat in Germany was 67:33, so that people ate twice as much rye as wheat. By 1970 it was already 25:75, meaning that three times as much wheat was eaten compared to rye. People are also eating much less bread altogether. In 1800, 300 kg of bread was eaten per head each year in Germany; by 1910 the figure had gone down to 157 kg, and by 1970 to 62 kg.

A look at the different grains

Wheat is the most widely grown grain in the world and is highly versatile. It can be used to make bread, cake, and the many delights for sale in pastry shops. It accommodates all different tastes (sweet, salty, or sour), especially if one uses highly refined white flour. It is easily digestible, has little flavor of its own, and provides a neutral base for any topping, whether it is butter, meat, cheese or jam that one actually wants. Thus, what was once 'our daily bread' has sunk to the level of a more or less tasteless base for spreading things on, and has little vitality. The same applies to snowy white rice: having no taste of its own, it makes an 'ideal' accompaniment for any kind of dish.

In recent years more and more people have been developing allergic reactions to milk and wheat, especially children with neurodermatitis. No doubt this is partly due to the fact that modern wheat is one-sided and that almost the only wheat bread eaten is baked with yeast. This modern wheat has been specially bred for its gluten content, that is, for proteins that give cohesiveness to the bread. The bread becomes soft and elastic. Thus, breeding does not focus on biological quality but on properties that are useful for baking technology. This qualitative change in the protein is probably the reason why more and more people have allergic reactions to wheat, for allergic reactions practically always have to do with proteins.

The extensive use of wheat in bread-baking in recent decades has a tragic aspect to it. Wheat is really the most refined and highly developed of all grains, and as always with something highly bred, it is not exactly robust and therefore not ideal for daily use. It seems that people had a sense for this in earlier times, for white bread and cake baked with wheat were eaten only on Sundays and festive occasions. They were mostly reserved for more well-to-do people, which was accepted in those days. On working days, of course, the heartier rye bread would be eaten.

The general way of thinking has changed completely since then. Everyone feels like a 'king' today, and all pleasures are available at any time, requiring as little effort as possible to obtain. People fail to notice that this is an illusory life style, lacking in moderation. We see this in the fate of wheat: this sun fruit, king of grains, Sunday food, has now been demoted to the status of a lowly servant for everyday use. To explain in what sense its biological value is not optimal, we might compare it to a concert pianist who is sent out to chop wood every day: the job will not get done very well, as the pianist's abilities lie in a very different direction. One might also say that there is no point in using a race horse (wheat) to pull a plow. The quality of the work would not only be poor, but the animal would be ruined in the process. Wheat that is misused in such a way cannot provide the right nourishment for people, and the body reacts with an allergy if misuse goes on for long enough.

This does not mean that wheat is 'bad'—quite the contrary! It is actually too precious for biological use only. In Old Testament times people had a feeling for this, for 'fine flour' (wheat) would only be used for rituals and at specific times. It was meant to be the basis for spiritual experience rather than biological life.

Specialization is always a problem, in the breeding of grains as much as with farm animals: cows bred and fed specifically to give high milk yields, pigs to put on meat, and chickens to be egg producers. The problem of all specialization is that high performance in one area always goes hand in hand with deficiency in another. Such high performance may lead to over-exploitation of the life forces and thus to susceptibility to diseases. Pedigree dogs are a good example. 'Mongrels' have much greater resistance to disease and are more robust, which means more vital. This is not to say anything against breeding as such, but that economic profit and high yields should not be the only criteria for breeding.

Spelt is an ancient variety of wheat that is not so overbred. It needs the special climate found primarily in the south of Germany and in Switzerland. A special characteristic of spelt is that it does not tolerate artificial fertilizer, or hardly at all, so that it is not possible to increase yields. Spelt harvested when milk-ripe and then dried in an oven is called *Grünkern* or 'green spelt.' It makes excellent tasty soups. Spelt bread is light and similar to wheat bread.

Rye is heartier, stronger tasting and 'heavier' than wheat. It has been the chief bread grain through the ages. But because of its strong taste, it is less suitable for cakes and pastries. In recent times people have tended to prefer an easier lifestyle and avoid effort of any kind. This means that they also prefer food which is easy to digest, especially sweets, none of which calls for any kind of digestive effort. Thus, bread manufacturers will often use wheat because it is lighter than rye, which is much more substantial. Many people hardly know the real taste of good, hearty bread anymore. Bread made with 100% rye is admittedly a bit too heavy for daily consumption. The ideal bread is rye bread lightened with 10-20% wheat. Rye prefers a rougher climate, which corresponds to its own nature, while wheat does well in milder, warmer regions.

Oats have the highest fat content of all grains (11%). This is why they quickly develop a bitter taste, showing that the fat in them has aged and grown rancid. Then they should not be eaten anymore. They also have a relatively high protein level, so that no other food needs to be added. Therefore, oats are generally used on their own in porridge, fried oat balls, and so on. Bread cannot be made out of oats. Diabetics in particular can profit from the combination of protein, fat and carbohydrates by having an 'oat day' once a week. On this day they eat only dishes made with oats instead of bread, potatoes, rice or other forms of carbohydrate. The relatively high fat content of oats does not elevate the cholesterol level; on the contrary, this fat stimulates bile excretion into the intestine. Thus the formation of new bile acid out of cholesterol is stimulated and the cholesterol level in the blood drops (see 'The Cholesterol Problem,' page 110). The outer husks of oats are extremely hard and special milling technology is required to remove them. It is a pity that the germ of the oat kernel is usually damaged in processing, causing the oats to lose the capacity to germinate, which means a loss of life forces. The grain is then rolled to produce oat flakes. Taken raw or cooked, these are a hearty universal food. But it is in the nature of things that rolled oats not only have lost the viability of their germ, but also can rarely ever be perfectly fresh by the time they reach the consumer, which means they have lost almost all of their life forces. That is why it is best to prepare oatmeal from freshly ground oats milled to a fine flour using oats that are capable of germinating, such as 'hulless' (or 'naked') oats. These are bred with loose husks so that the germ of the kernel is not damaged in processing. After grinding and soaking overnight, they can be cooked the next morning with a little salt and a dash of milk for five minutes, stirring continually. Then the porridge can be served with some cream or milk. These ground and soaked oats can also be eaten raw as raw grain muesli (see page 17) where they retain a maximum of vitality.

❧

Barley on its own, like oats, cannot be baked into bread. In antiquity it was the food of gladiators, who were called *hordearii*—'barley eaters.' Slaves were also fed barley. Both groups of people needed to be strong and capable of great physical effort. This shows that barley is one of the grains with the strongest life forces. A special feature of barley is that it has a high silica content. Humans need this mineral for their hair, skin, cartilage, bones and connective tissues. The ash of the outer parts of the grain contains up to 70% silica. Long awns are typical of barley. They act like antennae to receive cosmic influences which are then mediated by silica to act on connective tissues and the configuration of the whole body. Because silica relates strongly to light, as is revealed through the transparency of silica crystals, barley has also been called the 'arrow of light' (Gerbert Grohmann).[13] As part of nutrition, barley not only gives form to all connective tissue but also helps the sense organs and brain development.

Barley also has a high protein (10-15%) but a low fat content (2%). The whole grain without a hull is still used as pearl barley today. Hearty soups are made with this, especially in mountainous regions. As with oats, however, the husk of the barley must be removed, thus damaging the germ. But like naked oats, 'naked barley' is bred with a loose husk and keeps a viable germ, maintaining all of its life forces.

Today, barley is mainly used as animal feed and to produce malt. For the latter, barley is soaked until it germinates, then dried and coarsely milled. The resulting maltose (a sugar) is used together with beer yeast and hops to make beer.

'Barley water' also has a long tradition behind it. It is made by soaking the barley, boiling and then straining it and collecting the residual gelled material.* Even today it remains an excellent aid for colds, flus, fever, diseases affecting the mucous membranes (of the respiratory tract or stomach, in gastritis for instance) and for undernourishment.

If problems exist in the sphere of silica action—in hair, skin, cartilage, bones and connective tissue, and also in the sense organs—it may be helpful to make barley (and millet)

---

* 2 liters of cold water, 4 tablespoons of whole grain barley, 2 tablespoons of raisins, ½ teaspoon of cinnamon: Simmer 1½ hours, pass through a sieve, cool, and drink the strained gelled material throughout the day.

practically the only carbohydrate in the diet (instead of bread, potatoes, noodles or rice) for four weeks. This also helps with acne. Flaked or milled barley can be made into fried barley balls or porridge.

❧

Millet was a staple food of the poor for a long time. (Their food was sparse but healthy, while the rich were eating themselves sick. Today everyone is 'rich' where their food is concerned, and the situation has changed accordingly.) Millet is also rich in silica and can complement barley. It is cooked like rice and served with vegetables or meat. But millet can also be ground to meal, and like oats it can be eaten raw or cooked as porridge (see above). It is hardly suitable for eating raw when unground, nor is it good added to bread, as the baking temperature is not sufficient to make it edible and the bread tastes 'sandy.'

❧

These are the traditional cereal grains originating in Europe, while *rice* is 'at home' in the East. The way it grows already shows its nature, with every grain growing out of the water suspended freely on its private little stalk, as it were. The grain which comes closest to this is oats. Barley, too, is close to rice. In the West, on the other hand, *maize* (corn) is dominant. Unlike rice, its kernels are tightly pressed together on the cob. This plant has a much closer relationship to the earth—it is more 'earthbound.' Another characteristic of maize is that it is a greedy feeder, taking a lot out of the soil.

Through the differences between maize and rice, West and East, one can see how plants are shaped by their geographic situation. Having been consumed for millennia, they have also left their mark on the life style and mentality of people. In every respect, the European cereals occupy a middle position between these two extremes. Wheat, with the positive and negative aspects described, lies at the center.

Baking: Archetype of
Human Activity on Earth

It is not only the choice of fertilizers and the selection and mixture of grains which matter in baking bread, but also how the grain is processed. Insight and experience have shown that as far as possible, bread should be made out of the whole grain—that is, starch, hull and if possible germ, but not husk. The grain must be milled to a fine flour. Ideally flour is milled the day it is baked, because the grain is a living organism in itself. Aging starts as soon as the grain is milled, for this removes the protective layers and the separation between the germ and the starch. Enzymes needed for germination are released and can no longer serve that original purpose. Air (oxygen) gains access, and all this leads to chemical changes that ultimately mean aging, the fading away of life. After a while all that is left is energy in the form of calories. In order to get grain into an easily digestible form, a *fine* grinding of the whole grain is necessary. By no means can greater vitality be expected when whole unmilled grains are soaked and then used whole in baking to make 'whole grain' bread. And this bread is much more difficult to digest.

Feeding experiments on rats have shown that just 14 days after milling, the life in whole grain flour has been reduced to such a degree that a fourth generation fed on this flour, or on bread made with it, was no longer viable. In rats fed on freshly milled whole grain flour or bread made of it, the fourth generation suffered no harm. Therefore it is important to make the bread as soon as the grain has been milled to flour. We should add, however, that this holds true only for whole grain flour, for this alone contains those

* Likewise, the English word yeast must originally have referred to sourdough culture. Ed.

66

highly reactive (and living) substances! Highly refined white wheat flour will stay practically unchanged because the enzymes and vitamins of the outer layers have been removed. We might also say that white flour keeps better because it is dead, which also makes it very digestible. This is why in the USA, for instance, it is a legal requirement to add iron and vitamins to this 'bread' made with refined flour. As many (synthetic) vitamins as possible, minerals, trace elements and so on are added to get 'high quality' bread. The longer the list of additives, the 'better,' so it is believed. To top it off, a highly hardened fat is worked in, resulting in bread that is very soft and elastic—rather like styrofoam.

It seems that people in Europe are beginning to sense that white bread has no real quality. This is also why innumerable extras are added, producing not just a rye-wheat bread, but a four or six-grain bread with added nuts, flax seeds, sunflower seeds, pumpkin seeds, potato flour, soy, milk, raisins and many other things. None of these improve bread in the least. Millet too is an excellent grain, as already mentioned, but does not make better bread.

What is a sensible approach? Rye bread, being relatively heavy, can be lightened with a bit of wheat. However, potato flour does not belong in bread at all, as will become evident (see page 78). The addition of fats is also an 'achievement' of more recent times. As already mentioned, it makes the bread so soft that it hardly needs chewing—even not at all! Adding milk makes soft milk rolls, which are really more of a delicacy, i.e. more a mediator of pleasure than of life. Of course one cannot object to eating them on festive occasions and Sundays, but they are not at all for daily fare, or worse still for sole consumption.

The degree to which the flour is milled is important, that is, how much of the whole grain (starch, germ, and hull) is taken to make the flour. This results in the different 'types' of flour. How much of the hull is present in the flour is determined by the quantity of ash, i.e. minerals, left over after burning 100 grams of flour. The ash is then weighed. The starch in a grain contains only 0.4% ash, the hull about 5% ash. The higher the weight, the darker and heavier the flour, up to the point where the whole grain with all its hull has been milled. Flour containing 0.405% ash, for instance, is referred to as type 405. It is light in color and not much of the hull from the grain has been milled; almost only the starch has been used. Whole grain flours are above type 1000.

In earlier times, the original bread was made only out of flour and water—no other ingredients. Flour was mixed with water to bake flat bread. Its low water content made it keep well, but it also meant that it was hard. This is why it is hardly made any more today. Such ancient bread still exists in the form of crispbread (*Knäckebrot*), which can be made with the whole grain.

The usual method of baking bread is to let the dough 'rise.' Bubbles of carbon dioxide gas loosen it up. Carbon dioxide is a break-down product of lactobacilli and, above all, of yeast. The resulting bread has many small holes in it, which makes it easier to chew and digest.

For thousands of years sourdough was used to make dough rise. There is evidence that this method was already used in ancient Egypt and has been known all over the world. Thus it cannot have been a chance discovery, as it is 'explained' today, but must have been developed from profound insight into the workings of nature. The souring happens because air always contains lactobacilli. As already described, when these get into milk they break down the milk sugar (lactose) to lactic acid (lactate), and under suitable conditions will also thrive in the starch of the dough. Rye is a much more favorable nutrient base for the lactobacilli than wheat. Rye flour stirred with water and kept at about 30°C turns into sourdough in about three days. To make absolutely certain that the process is working, a little sour milk or whey can be added. This relatively small amount of sourdough is then worked into the total amount of dough used for baking. A small amount of the sourdough (the 'starter') is always be kept back and stored in a cool place for the next baking. It is then added to the new dough, thus passing on the lactobacilli (technically, 'inoculating' the dough). This method takes time and is sensitive to changes in temperature and even to the influence of the weather.

This natural fermentation produces mainly lactic acid in the bread, but depending on the 'direction' given it also produces carbon dioxide, acetic acid and other products which give the bread its typical aromatic taste. Higher temperatures promote the production of acetic acid, while more moderate heat favors lactic acid production. Natural sourdough is not a uniform substance but a living organism that adapts to the nutrient base and environmental conditions—just as yeasts do in wine making. This has already been considered in detail. It is the same principle as with sour milk, salt cucumbers and sauerkraut production. Let it be stressed once again that this breaking down of carbohydrates to lactic acid is wholly in harmony with human metabolism, in which sugar is broken down to lactic acid and not to alcohol. The traditional method of baking with sourdough is very time-consuming and is really an art. Time costs money nowadays, and so 'quick souring' and 'artificial souring methods' have been developed. They miss the point, however, for it is not the end product that matters, but the signaling of which direction to take. An even quicker method is simply to add vinegar or some other acid to bread, but this completely misses the point of baking.

A less familiar way of baking is the preparation of 'honey-salt bread,' which originated in the Mazdaznan movement and was mentioned by Rudolf Steiner.

Following the idea of honey-salt bread, a starter dough was developed with the addition of legume flour. This then led to the development of *Backferment* ('baking enzyme'). It consists of specially bred highly active lactobacilli and yeasts. This product is very practical for simple household use because the bread always turns out well. (In older times it was a farmer's secret to add pea flour to the dough in order to give the bread good consistency and cohesiveness.) With the *Backferment*, even grains not suitable for baking can be used for bread making (for instance, corn and buckwheat), a fact which can be useful for those suffering from celiac disease. But because *Backferment* bread contains more yeast than sourdough, it is less healthy than sourdough bread. (See 'The Problem of Using Yeast in Baking,' page 71.)

The Problem of
Using Yeast in Baking

The old German word *hevo* ('lifting substance, leavening'), from which the modern German word *Hefe* ('yeast') derives, has existed for more than 1000 years. But *hevo* did not mean what we call yeast today. That word undoubtedly referred to sourdough and not to yeast, because yeast was only discovered in 1854 when Pasteur, working with alcoholic fermentation, found that yeast is required for it. It 'lifts' the fluid by generating gas (carbon dioxide). The name *hevo*, known from bread making since the medieval times, was then applied to these isolated organisms.* Much later they were classified under the fungi, subclass yeasts. Later followed further differentiation of the yeasts used in beer brewing and it became possible to isolate baker's yeast from beer yeast and produce it industrially.

In recent decades the original method of using sourdough to make bread has been almost completely superseded by the use of yeast. The reason is the saving of time, as mentioned, and above all that baking with yeast calls for no special skill. Everyone is certain to succeed. However, this also means that the body is shown another path of breaking down carbohydrates. This is the direction of *alcoholic fermentation*, which is not in accord with human nature.

Of course, no one will suffer harm from eating a white roll baked with yeast. However, if this becomes the only 'bread' many people eat for generations, then carbohydrate breakdown will be directed improperly. The described consequences will then have to follow. (See 'Understanding Digestive Functions,' page 51)

In nature, yeasts are found on the skins of sweet fruit. They are literally sitting there waiting to fall upon their real life element, sugar. Sugars and yeast are very close to one another,

71

comparable to the relationship between protein and putrefying bacteria. The metabolism of these microbes differs from that of humans.

There is, however, one exception: the lactobacilli. These 'belong' to milk and rye just as yeasts belong to sugar and wheat. They are also able to break down sugar, but in a very different way from yeasts, doing it exactly the same way humans break down sugar—to lactic acid. Bread can be baked with lactobacilli (sourdough) just as well as with added yeast. The difference is that the ways of breaking down the sugar are completely different. Yeasts produce alcohol as well as carbon dioxide. This does not mean that yeast-baked bread contains enough alcohol to cause inebriation. Alcohol has a much lower boiling point than water and evaporates more or less completely during baking. The important point is rather that the breaking down of sugar or starch is taken in another *direction* with yeast than it is with sourdough. In the human organism, the breaking down of sugar must not produce alcohol but lactic acid.

A problem thus arises that no one recognizes today. How does bread baked with natural sourdough act on human beings compared to the 'same' bread—that is, the same dough—baked with yeast? As already stated, baking—and the grinding of flour which precedes it—breaks down the grain in a kind of predigestion. The organism follows the direction which is given to it. And the directions of yeast and lactobacilli are very different. Lactic acid, produced in the sourdough process, is wholly in accord with the human metabolism. People were clearly aware of this in earlier times, for they used this procedure all over the world with different kinds of products (bread, sauerkraut, salted cucumbers, kvass). The breaking down to alcohol is not at all in accord with human metabolism, even if small traces of alcohol may arise in human metabolism. The special properties of lactic acid have been fully discussed in the respective chapter (see page 28).

The problem lies not so much in the products which arise (the lactic acid that remains in bread or the alcohol that escapes in baking), as more importantly in the predisposition that is set for the further direction to be followed in breaking down substances.

Of course, human beings are able to change a direction which is presented to them or which they have initially taken. The problem lies in the long-term effect, which is the general problem with nutrition. Just 100 years ago, yeast started to be used not only for beer brewing but also for baking. Its use has continued to grow to the point that today bread is almost always baked with yeast. No one questions this anymore and it is simply assumed that this is what 'bread' is. However, what this means is that the human metabolism has now been programmed in a different direction for generations, starting in earliest childhood.

One has to understand that baker's yeast as such does no harm. On the contrary, it is an excellent provider of vitamin B. After all, it consists of selectively bred, pure yeast cells. We have to realize, however, that all microorganisms, be they bacteria, yeasts, fungi or viruses, are extremely versatile and adaptable. They will quickly adapt to a suitable environment, changing both the environment and themselves. For instance, the yeast in bread can easily transform into intestinal yeast.

An added problem is that sugar consumption, as mentioned before, has also steadily increased over the last 150 years.[8] Sugar, of course, is the ideal nutrient base for yeasts, unless it is highly concentrated as in jam. Sweet fruits offer yeasts the right environment on their surfaces, while milk, rye and vegetables provide a natural growth environment for the lactic-acid-producing lactobacilli.

It is easy to see, therefore, that both increased sugar consumption and the 'misguided' breaking down of flour in the intestines create ideal conditions for yeasts. The result is a medical problem which is increasingly causing concern:

yeast infections. The wild forms of yeast are often 'stronger' than the lactobacilli, but the human organism is still able to cope with this. The more important point is not only that people ingest great quantities of yeast along with the bread they eat and provide it with the ideal nutrient base through high sugar and white wheat flour consumption, but that this consumption points in the wrong direction—that of yeast rather than lactobacilli fermentation. However, the effects are not immediately apparent. They take decades to reveal themselves. This is a question of learning! Every child must learn, when weaned, to cope with foods which are at first unfamiliar, such as cow's milk and grains. The child will gradually move to stronger foods. If a child does not learn to make the necessary effort and develop the ability to digest, the metabolism will remain weak. Eventually there will be many things that the child can no longer digest. Sugar, white bread and similar foods encourage this development, as they make no demands on the organism, as shown previously. If at the same time the human organism is shown a direction for breaking down starch—not just for years but for decades and generations—that is anything but what it should be, taking the direction of the yeast towards alcohol rather than sourdough towards lactic acid, and doing so daily, then the organism learns to select this wrong direction. This changes the whole constitution. The consequence is that the yeasts, which depend on this direction, will multiply and grow stronger. They will finally colonize not only the intestine but also other organs, such as the vagina or lung.

If these 'yeasts gone wild' (above all *Candida*) would simply produce alcohol like 'respectable' yeasts, it would not be so terrible—and it does happen. What is much more dangerous is that these wild yeasts not only spread uninhibitedly but may degenerate further and produce substances comparable to 'rotgut,' low-toxicity fatty acids, and many other things that do not belong in the human metabolism. The same may happen in wine-making, with cheap wines, when fermentation has not been properly guided. The result will be hangover (headache, nausea, and so on). It is not only the intestine which is upset, therefore; the above-mentioned metabolic products will also affect the liver as well as the immune system and even mood levels.

The fact that sugar plays a major role in all of this is known today. Unfortunately cutting down only on sugar will no longer solve the problem; those affected must avoid *every kind* of sweet and sweetening agent, white flour products and yeast-baked bread, as well as the skin of fruits ('anti-yeast diet'). Most patients are only prepared to put up with this when they have tried everything else and reached the limit of their endurance.

There are, of course, highly effective drugs that will kill the yeasts. In most cases they will give marked improvement, but the original problem will soon return when the sufferer stops using the antimycotics. Therefore, apart from the above-mentioned sugar-free diet, it is necessary to use an oral treatment to improve the intestinal flora. Many preparations are available with specially bred, highly powerful intestinal bacteria that will suppress the yeast. Also charcoal, ideally made from coffee beans, will detoxify. In addition, all bitters stimulate the function of the digestive organs. It is important to continue such treatments for a long period (6-12 months). After all, the degeneration of the metabolism and the yeast growth did not develop in just a few days.

Of course, other factors also play a role here. It is known today that antibiotics kill not only the pathogenic bacteria but also, and more likely, the 'friendly' bacteria in the intestine, among them the lactobacilli—but not the yeasts. People are realizing only now that antibiotics, the 'miracle drug,' have been much too generously prescribed. Many of the preservatives, colorants, emulsifiers and disinfectants (e.g. in toothpaste) which are often quite unnecessarily added to products also do not have positive effects on the intestinal flora with long-term use. Emotional factors can also affect intestinal function, as people have known for ages. The intestine mirrors the state of the soul. Food, however, remains the main factor affecting the intestine and/or causing the intestinal flora to degenerate. In the long run, this phenomenon of 'going wild' (not only of yeasts, but quite generally of bacteria, viruses and even insects, as well as the progressive 'going wild of the soul') calls for reflection on the fundamentals of our way of life and the need for change—in our nutrition too.

In earlier times when people still felt their work to be meaningful, they knew that the food they ate influenced how they experience the spiritual. In the Old Testament, careful distinction is therefore made between *leavened* (soured) bread and *unleavened* (unsoured) flat bread, which probably referred to wheat. Daily bread intended for earthly activity was, of course, soured. For offerings, however, it was specially stated that this should be 'unleavened (...) cakes of fine flour (...) and unleavened flat breads' (Numbers 6,15). 'No grain offering which you present to the Lord shall be made with leaven' (Leviticus 2,11). The earth influence which comes with souring is not meant to enter into flour that is still 'purely cosmic.' This applied to the days of 'unleavened bread' during Passover, a period of offering during which people were to avoid connecting with earthly activities and so be open to spiritual cosmic processes. The New Testament as well expressly advises keeping such customs (Luke 22,7; Acts 12,3). Until a few decades ago these things survived in central Europe as tradition. Thus, people would eat white bread only on Sundays or festive occasions. During the week dark rye bread made with sourdough would be brought to the table. There is no need to be fanatical about these old customs, but the wholesale change to eating white bread made of wheat and yeast has influenced the human metabolism, as we have seen, though people do not yet realize it. The change in bread-eating habits reflects the modern attitude of treating every day as if it were Sunday.

Summing up, one may say that bread should really be a fundamental part of human nutrition. But most modern breads are far removed from the ideal. What matters is not only the kind of grain used, its provenance, and the methods of soil fertilization and harvesting, but above all the steps that follow: the grinding and the baking. These are almost completely industrialized today and fail to serve a deeper purpose. The point of baking is not simply to make digestion easier; it is human labor that *takes further* the food nature has given. Appropriate *hand*ling brings bread closer to human nature, going beyond the merely biological aspect of supporting life. It should serve to connect us to the earth in a *human* way. Properly guided mildly *de*structive processes such as souring can initiate a new *con*structive process. In this respect, the original bread-baking process offers an archetypal image for the meaning of human work on earth.

Bread and vegetables are the natural source of carbohydrates. In the 18th century, however, the *potato* was brought to Europe from Central America and now forms a large element in the diet. An understanding of its influence on human beings will not be evident from its 'composition' of starch, protein and other ingredients. Its origin and manner of growth do, however, reveal what is important about the potato. Grains always grow and ripen at the highest point of the plant. Many of the vegetables we eat come from the leaf or root (cauliflower is, of course, a 'flower'). This gives some indication as to their use as food. In the spiritual scientific view of the human being, roots relate to the human head and nervous system. Therfore when these need strengthening, vitalizing and supporting, preference should be given to roots. (The fact that horseradish is active in the head region can be a direct experience.) Like roots, potatoes grow below ground, yet they are not roots but tubers which derive from the stem. Therefore by nature their proper place is *above* ground. It is always a problem if something grows in the 'wrong' place. It is also plain to see that true roots are highly formed, whereas potatoes do not really have a proper form. The processes which create form come from the light. This can be seen when plants grow with little light; they are pale and grow tall with less form. For humans, this means that potato tubers, pretending to be roots, inevitably have effect in the sphere of the nerves but lack the power of form that should accompany this. With long-term use, the lack of form will affect the whole body. This is visible in the big belly people get when they eat a lot of potatoes, which is popularly called 'potato belly' (*Kartoffelbauch*) in German. What is more important, this effect can also extend to our thinking, for to think is to live in the light. This does not mean that eating potatoes makes people stupid—rather the contrary. A thinking that is more or less lacking in light will extend particularly to earthly things, for instance the technological thinking which is so highly developed today.

It is also important to be aware that the potato belongs to the nightshade family (Solanaceae). All plants in that family are poisonous in one way or another. Some, like tobacco or deadly nightshade (atropa belladonna), are poisonous in all parts. Others produce the poison only in some of their parts. Potato does so in the fruit, for instance, but not in the tuber. The tubers can also produce poison, however, if exposed to light so that they turn green. Other members of the nightshade family, such as tomato, aubergine (eggplant), and sweet pepper, have non-poisonous fruits and may therefore be eaten. Again there is nothing to be said against eating potatoes or tomatoes, provided it is done in 'suitable moderation.' In various regions people have gone far beyond the limits of moderation. Many vegetables have been practically pushed aside by tomatoes, aubergines and sweet peppers. This again creates one-sidedness.

Meat or Vegetarian?

Is it best to keep to a purely vegetarian diet, or does meat deserve a place on the menu? This question has been a subject of lively dispute for many years. On the one hand there is evidence that in order to survive, humans need certain amino acids that occur only in meat. The conclusion is that man cannot live without meat. On the other hand there are people who have never eaten meat, and they remain healthy—in fact more healthy than meat eaters. There is statistical proof to show this. Nevertheless, both types of diet will continue to be advocated as 'the only right one.' What is behind this?

Those who follow a vegetarian diet take no meat but will eat milk, milk products, eggs and fish, although the situation is not entirely clear with regard to fish. Many therefore like to speak of a 'lacto-vegetarian diet,' which includes milk products and plants.

What is so special about meat? Why is it that vegetarians refuse to eat meat but not milk and milk products?

Some people have a natural aversion to meat. Others argue that if people had to kill the chicken or the calf themselves, they would instantly turn vegetarian.

Meat is muscle tissue from an animal, including the heart. Various internal organs such as liver, lung, thymus and stomach were also eaten in earlier times. Today only muscle is called 'meat.'

In the past people knew full well what meat really signifies. The process in which the spirit or soul unites with the body was called 'incarnation,' which means 'entering into the flesh.' The text of the Latin Mass still says '*et incarnatus est.*' People were very much aware then that the human being lives in the flesh, and above all in the heart. Today hardly anyone questions the assumption that the seat of the soul (i.e. the psyche) is the brain; it is just taken for granted. Yet in reality the seat of the soul is the flesh.

This means, however, that meat from a chicken, pig or cow contains not only life, but that a part of the animal's soul nature is incarnated in it. The biological effect of eating meat is not as important as the effect of the soul element of the animal which is connected with the meat. This does not mean, of course, that people who eat lots of chicken will gradually turn into chickens. Nevertheless, they will take a little of the 'animal quality' into themselves with the meat. We can see the truth of this when we study people who consume great amounts of meat. They are more lively, impulsive, and sometimes even more aggressive. A genuine study of the human being will recognize that these qualities are completely independent of the biological value of the food. The latter is of course the basis on which a soul can unfold. Biological life must be there. But it is a totally different question whether it is also imbued with soul qualities.

The difference becomes even more apparent when one meets people who do not eat *anything* that comes from animals. They do not take eggs, milk or milk products. These are vegans, the strictest kind of vegetarians. People who adhere to this life style for decades will show definite changes. Some of the above-mentioned characteristics such as aggressiveness or excessively emotional reactions will lie quite outside their range of behavior. Some nutrition experts say that such people grow remote from life or indeed are unable to deal with life. It may seem like this in our times, but it will be permitted to ask: Is today's emphatically aggressive life style more supportive of life? More in harmony with life? The influence of nutrition extends to social life.

These examples show that meat has a stimulating effect on the human soul. Meat-eating generally makes people more wide-awake. How someone uses this wakefulness is quite another matter. This is a matter of the spirit.

It may be objected that following a big meal of meat one is more tired than after a vegetable platter. This observation is correct. However, what we are speaking of here is not the immediate effect but only the effects after months, perhaps even years or decades—that is, the influence on the constitution.

In today's way of looking at things, where the focus is one-sidedly on physical substances, the difference between meat and milk products such as cheese tends to be blurred. It is said that after all, both are simply protein and fat. This is a gross over-simplification and misses the reality. What was just said about meat does not in fact apply at all to milk and its products. Meat and blood are red, milk is white. This alone should speak volumes. For people who retain a feeling for color, red is still today a sign of warmth, but also of stimulation and even aggressiveness. White is neutral and soothing. Of course, the difference may also be 'explained' in chemical terms. Blood contains iron, which gives it its red color. Milk gets its white color from the fat emulsified in it; that is, fat is evenly distributed as very small droplets in the milk's watery part. The fat particles do not let the light through but reflect it, producing the white color. In addition, milk has extremely low iron levels. Infants, for whom milk is intended, are not meant to be active, let alone hyperactive. They should be quietly growing. This applies to the young until puberty. Many members of the medical profession do not realize this today, and iron is added to many milk products for babies, although it has no effect because it is excreted.

Milk contains a highly sensitive and unstable protein. It does not contain the animal's soul component, which is in the meat. Meat of any kind is therefore unsuitable for young children, and even less so for babies.

With older children, on the other hand, it may sometimes be necessary to give meat. Especially girls who tend to be a bit sleepy or slow often have a real craving for meat or sausage. If they are allowed to have these, in just a few weeks one may see them becoming more 'awake' and developing more in accord with their age. We may, of course, 'explain' this by saying that meat—again in contrast to milk—contains more of the phosphorus and iron which the child 'needs.' In any case, this is a completely individual problem and has to do with the child's constitution. But it should be evident that meat consumption has increased so much today that children's constitutions are being altered accordingly, or even ruined. Meat is definitely not a generally needed basic food. It is more of a stimulant, a mediator of pleasure, which is why consumption is rising.

A look at the main types of meat

As already mentioned, meat contains something of the animal's soul nature. Thus it is understandable why most humans are not accustomed to eating cats or dogs, at least not in the usual run of things. (In China dog meat is considered a delicacy, but not 'normal' (everyday) meat. It has been mentioned that dogs and cats live principally on other animals. Their meat would thus be of inferior biological value. But there is a soul element in addition. Cats and dogs are predators by nature. If people were to eat such meat in large quantities or for long periods (decades or generations), something of this soul quality would pass on to them. Humans have therefore from time immemorial rejected the meat of carnivores. (Eskimos appear to be an exception. They eat seal, for instance, which live on fish. It must be considered, however, that their conditions of life are substantially different and cannot simply be applied to other life styles.)

꙳

Beef: In comparing a cow with a dog or a cat, the difference is immediately evident. The slightly dim, dreamy look in the eye, the heaviness and slowness—all this speaks of a creature that is self-contained and at peace. (In India, where the cow is held sacred, people are still clearly aware of this.) But for those who are not vegetarians, beef is therefore the ideal form of meat.

❧

Pork: In recent decades increasing amounts of pork have been produced, recommended and eaten. Nobody seems to find this strange. Pork is said to be rich in protein, low in fat (thanks to modern breeding methods), high in vitamin B, and so forth. This may be correct but misses the point. Meat consumption as a whole has gone down slightly since 1994, but in 2009 pork was still the most consumed meat in Germany, accounting for 64% of total per-person meat consumption (39 kg pork out of 60 kg total meat consumption).

Jews and Muslims, on the other hand, avoid pork for religious reasons. This ban goes back to times when religion permeated all spheres of life. These peoples—and many others—had religious rules that extended to medicine, nutrition and hygiene. The question is why, more than 3,000 years ago, a taboo was put particularly on the hog (in fact on animals which have split hooves and are not ruminants). Modern people believe the 'explanation' to be that pigs are dirty—a view which is both superficial and wrong. Pigs will by nature root in the soil to find their food. That they get dirty doing this is natural. However, observing a family of pigs in a sty built to meet their needs, one finds that they use one corner for defecation, have a separate sleeping area, and are not at all dirty. But they do in fact eat everything, including meat. This raises the matter discussed above, namely that humans should not eat carnivores.

More important is the fact that domesticated pigs are closer to humans than other animals (even than apes) in that they are the only animals that are naked. This is not something superficial but an expression of their nature! The arrangement of their teeth also corresponds quite exactly to that of humans, though they are bigger in size. All other mammals show distinct specialization of teeth. They develop either the molars, the canines, or the incisors. But in humans and in pigs, all three types of teeth are equally developed. What is more, it has been found that the metabolic organs (kidney, liver, heart) of pigs are startlingly similar to those of humans.

Attempts are therefore in progress to transplant porcine hearts and livers into humans when human organs are not available. This is already being done successfully with porcine heart valves. That it can already be done, and in the future may be done on a large scale, only shows that human beings have lost all feeling for the nature of life, soul and spirit.

One might argue that this very similarity should make pork good for humans. In an odd way this is true, but only to a certain degree. Pork is easily digested. This, however, is where the problem lies. Pig protein is relatively similar to human protein. It is therefore not only easily broken down, but for this very reason it is hardly recognized as foreign by the metabolism of some people. It is therefore not broken down sufficiently and taken up in a 'half' broken-down state. Everyone who suffers from a rheumatic condition will probably know this from experience: their condition worsens the day after eating a fairly large amount of pork. This is because the pork is reabsorbed before it has been completely broken down. The organism must then defend itself against it on the inside, that is, in the muscles or joints. Painful inflammation results as it tries to break down the foreign protein.

Again one is tempted to say that this only applies to people with rheumatic conditions. But through them light is thrown on the whole situation. Once again, a healthy person will not suffer harm from eating moderate amounts of pork. Excessive consumption, however—not to speak of unbroken pork consumption over thousands of years—can indeed change the human constitution. It is not that people get 'piggish,' but that this animal principle, too close to that of humans, may undermine our constitution. This was revealed to the leaders of humanity thousands of years ago.

Except for people with rheumatic conditions, healthy individuals should have no problem eating pork today, with one condition, however: The quantity eaten should be the same as in former times. Every farm used to keep just enough pigs to eat and consume the organic wastes. Food was considered a gift of God, something not to be thrown out as is done today. Then once a year a pig would be killed. Today, pork consumption is many times greater. In the long run therefore, this level of consumption must have an influence—especially on the metabolic system, which will grow weaker. This in turn will affect other spheres, including our natural defenses, weakening the immune system. Unfortunately the term 'immune deficiency' is chiefly associated with AIDS today, which is a misleading oversimplification. In reality human defenses against, or resistance to, external influences are decreasing all over the world. This is clearly evident in the tremendous increase in allergic diseases.[6]

❧

Chickens are birds and as such are more remote from humans than mammals. By nature they live in the air and do not connect fully with the earth. Their meat, the carrier of their nature, is therefore also 'lighter,' a bit more cosmic. Until quite recently it was therefore generally known that chicken stock was an excellent restorative, especially for anyone recovering from an illness. The stock does not contain meat but the extract of it. Convalescents would later on be given chicken meat to help them recover. This custom came from ancient knowledge of the animal's nature. Today it is no longer true to the same extent. Chickens are largely raised on an industrial scale and not in a way that meets their needs. People increasingly realize that keeping laying hens in cages and raising chickens in huge numbers only to fatten them is not in accord with the animal's true nature. Yet even animal breeders who realize this and are willing to do it differently find it difficult to survive in competition with the highly rationalized, high-yield industrial concerns which offer their products at extremely low prices.

This applies generally and has to be taken into account. In animal husbandry, just as with field crops, concern for biological needs is sacrificed to the principle of economic profitability. Pigs are bred for meat but their muscular development is stunted, indeed impossible in narrow confinement. This meat comes from an organ of movement that has not been developed.

✢

Veal is more tender than beef and therefore can be sold at a better price. Producers will try to keep the calves as calves for as long as possible. The young calves are separated from the mothers at an early age and kept in dark stalls or hutches. A diet deficient in iron is supplied to make the animals anemic, and this keeps the meat pale. This 'calf,' which in the meantime will have reached quite a size, is fed nothing but a liquid diet. This is dried milk from surpluses (generally skimmed milk powder) mixed with water. The milk from the calves' own mothers is sold, or the cows may become pregnant again and therefore 'go dry,' as farmers say.

From what has been said, it should not be difficult to see that the animal's soul, the influence of which extends to its protein, will have an influence also in these products. The evident cruelty of keeping and killing animals in ways that are not in accord with their natural needs must enter into the product. Again it must be emphasized that influences like these will not be immediately apparent. They will show themselves years later if these things continue to be ignored.

❧

Fish meat is in a class of its own. Fish are even more distant from humans than birds. We see this from their whole way of life. The latter may vary enormously, however: from trout that strive toward the source of the light-filled stream, to deep-sea fish that live in darkness and can develop frightful appearances. In between are the actual saltwater fish which humans have been catching and eating through the ages. Many of them are out-and-out predators, living on other fish. Here the food chain concept comes into play which we developed earlier—that biological life decreases in repeated passages. Yet it does not apply so much in the case of fish, as they live in sea water which is full of vitality. The sea is really the reservoir of life on earth. Fish do not have the same degree of conscious awareness as do terrestrial animals, an awareness that depends on destructive processes. Their vitality expresses itself in an enormous capacity to reproduce. One fish produces many hundreds of eggs.

Practically all saltwater fish produce vitamins A and D. Halibut and cod have particularly high levels of these. As cod liver oil, its fat has pronounced healing properties, above all because of high levels of vitamin A and unsaturated fatty acids. It has recently been discovered that *cold*-water sea fish such as mackerel, herring and salmon produce a particularly health-giving and highly active oil which is used to dissolve deposits formed in blood vessels, above all in dementia and heart disease.

Compared to saltwater fish, trout—raised nowadays mainly in ponds—lack the above-mentioned fats. They depend almost one hundred percent on factory-made food and therefore have to be specially treated before killing to improve their taste. Their protein is therefore more of a delicacy than a healthy food.

An exception to the healthfulness of sea fish is found in crustaceans (cray fish, crabs, lobsters, and so forth). They eat animals that eat animals, which means that the life in them is not just second-hand, but third or fourth-hand. What is even more problematic, they mostly eat *dead* animals. This means that crustaceans not only have little life force, they also have a dubious soul quality. This is why Jews and Muslims have banned crustaceans from their diet.

In the New Testament, the feeding of the five thousand is done with bread and fishes. This is given as an image. Evidently fish, like bread, can be a carrier of cosmic impulses, and these cosmic impulses are what truly matter.

~&

It is known today that excessive amounts of protein may cause chronic poisoning. Recommended amounts have been greatly reduced in recent times, since on the whole people are eating much too much protein. Nevertheless, materialistic thinking repeatedly asserts itself. Since most of the substance in the human and animal body consists of protein, it is thought that much protein is needed to build and maintain it, and that vegetarians could easily suffer protein deficiency. But a purely vegetarian animal such as a cow makes it clear that this is not the case. A cow consists of hundreds of kilograms of protein and also produces a large amount of protein in its milk every day and yet eats nothing but plants. Obviously the *buildup* of protein is independent of the *intake* of protein. But people still worry about a possible protein deficiency in their food.

Therefore many people, not only vegetarians, look for a *vegetable* protein—a protein that comes from plants—to replace animal protein. This they find in *mushrooms*. The consumption of mushrooms has increased enormously in recent years. Just a few decades ago, people would only eat mushrooms in the season when they grow, in late summer and fall. New methods have made it possible to grow mushrooms at any time and in ways that make collection easy.

What is the nature of mushrooms? They grow in pastures and woods but they are not green. This means they have no chlorophyll and therefore do not live on light. Light even impedes their development. Mushrooms are therefore grown in cellars in complete darkness. This is where the problem arises. The mushroom only pretends to be a plant! It is not really a plant, because a 'proper' plant lives on sunlight. Mushrooms need food that is decomposing, food that is losing its life. This is why mushrooms are often grown on horse manure in the dark. Their body substance is protein, i.e. of animal nature, although they behave like plants. They produce protein, which is by nature completely without light. Plants produce carbohydrates, which are essentially condensed light, as we have shown in the early chapters. Again, it is not their composition which matters—amino acids, vitamins, and so on—but the fact that mushroom substance is lightless protein. Of course it can be eaten and processed by the body, but its qualitative influence is not in accord with the process of life. As a matter of fact, this protein is the same as the protein formed by insects (chitin). Again, this is not to say that one should never eat mushrooms. It becomes a matter of concern, however, that in recent decades mushrooms are added to almost every meat dish and in the USA *raw* mushrooms are often added to salads. This introduces a qualitative element of *lightlessness* into the organism which must in the long run have a negative influence, though less so in the biological than in the soul sphere.

Certainly not directly, but indirectly this type of metabolism also supports the growth of other 'mushrooms' (i.e. fungi), namely the yeasts. Thus it encourages the many 'yeast infections' which were discussed above (pages 73-74).

In their search for a plant protein, people also turn to soybeans. Beans in general belong to the legume family, which is characteried by high protein formation in contrast to 'proper' plants which typically form carbohydrates. This fact already indicates that legume behavior is contrary to the true nature of plants. In the Pythagorean academy beans were not eaten, because at that time their intake hindered sharp, logical thinking. Today the human constitution is such that beans no longer have much of an influence on thinking, but only on our digestion, generating gas. The knowledge that eating beans could dull the thinking is reflected in the German expression 'He has wind in his head.' In fact beans, especially soybeans, contain a substance (phasin) that inhibits some digestive enzymes, which is why they are hard to digest. This substance is destroyed by heat treatment and also partly by sprouting, so soybeans must always be cooked or sprouted before eating. But the fact that they have a negative effect in the raw state reveals something about their nature that should be taken into consideration in seeking a healthy diet.

Eggs: Concentrated Life

Eggs are inexpensive today and may be bought in large amounts at any time. Until just a few decades ago eggs were available only in spring, when the hens were laying. People, being so clever, have of course changed this by keeping laying hens in confined spaces exposed to artificial light for many hours a day. The hens are thus put under production stress.

What is an egg, really? The shape of it will tell someone who attends to these things that it is practically the opposite of a crystal. Crystals with their exact facets exist only in the non-living world, while the shape of the egg exists only in the living world. The egg is the typical shape of life—we might also say a typical form of the cosmos. This may sound unusual, but it is so. Every educated person has learned that the earth and the other planets move around the sun in circular orbits. Of course, this is not quite accurate, for they actually move in ellipses—the shape of an egg! Even the earth, often pictured as round, is not exactly round. If we cut it in half, we would see that it, too, is elliptical (a rotation ellipsoid, to be precise). The ellipse and the egg are cosmic shapes. This shape protects new life from earthly influences coming in at the wrong time. It makes it possible for cosmic forces to enter, in this case life. For life comes in from the cosmos with the sun's light.

An egg is a complete organism. This is why a new organism, the chick, can come from it. This process has been fully investigated. The future chick develops from the yellow egg yolk. Therefore it should be evident that egg yolk contains life in concentrated form, in this case 'ensouled' life. People knew this in the past and to some extent still do. One or two raw egg yolks would be combined with a little honey and red wine and given to convalescents. But this was not given to really

91

sick patients, since these must use their forces to overcome the disease. The digestion of an egg would be an additional burden. But convalescents have some free forces again and can now benefit from egg yolk's great vitality. That vitality of the yolk is lost in a hardboiled egg, but is still present in a raw or soft boiled egg.

It was also known that the concentrated life in the egg is *ensouled* life, since eggs were once used as an aphrodisiac. Nowadays, eggs are also given to young children. This is well meant, but it introduces a foreign vitalization for which the child is not ready at this stage. The whole digestive organism of a young child will only be more or less ready to cope with such a food from about the age of three years on. Eating too many eggs in puberty is also a problem. The kind of 'ensouled' vitality which this introduces can lead to excessive sexuality, something young people at this age already have enough problems dealing with.

Average egg consumption is undoubtedly much higher today than a century ago. It is doubtful, however, whether their vitality is still the same, considering the industrial methods used to keep and feed animals nowadays.

In recent years we have heard insistent warnings against eating eggs, especially the yolk, due to their relatively high cholesterol content. We shall consider this in detail later.

The Various Fats and Their Effects

For most of history, food rich in fat was always considered to be good food because fat satisfies more intensively and longer than protein or carbohydrates. This can be quantified today. Both protein and carbohydrates have a 'nutrient value' of 4.1 calories per gram, compared to 9.3 calories for fat, which is more than twice as much.

It has been mentioned that plants consist largely of carbohydrates and that the living substance of animals and humans is protein. Fat is present in both and thus occupies a middle position.

Fat is a food and therefore contains life, but it must also have something special which the other two lack. What is the nature of fat? A clue may be found in the way plants produce fats. Roots are all practically fat-free, leaves contain very little fat, but *all* seeds contain oil, a liquid fat. What is the nature of a seed? It stores the concentrated life of the plant. This will only emerge again when the plant germinates a year or more later. Seeds develop in the fruits which follow the flowers, and are generally found in the uppermost parts of the plant. These parts are therefore exposed to the most intense cosmic light. This in itself shows that fats do not belong to the earth. Fats are in fact lighter than carbohydrates or protein and even lighter than water. This means they transcend at least the region of water, which is the sphere of life. Only exceptional plants produce fats also in their fruits, such as the olive, the avocado and the coconut.

There is one exception: the peanut. It ripens in the *soil*, which is why it is called the 'earthnut' (*Erdnuss*) in German. This is unusual. It clearly goes against the nature of plants and expresses itself even in the chemistry of peanut oil.

Again, this does not mean that we should not use peanut oil. It is very thin and not highly active, so that it hardly turns rancid and is thus suitable for external uses such as massage oil, for example, but not for nourishment.

All animals produce fats, higher animals in specific fatty tissues. Generally speaking animal fats are more solid than liquid vegetable oils, which means they melt at a higher temperature. But these things depend largely on the exterior temperature. Plants growing in colder regions produce oils with low melting points (e.g. flaxseed oil). In the tropics, on the other hand, plants produce harder fats with much higher melting points (e.g. coconut oil).

The same happens in the animal world. If we compare the fat of sheep in the warm climate of southern Spain with that of sheep in the north of England, for instance, we find that the southern sheep fat has a significantly higher melting point. The same relationship is shown by the following experiment. One group of young pigs was kept at 30°C to 35°C, another at 0°C. The melting point of the fat from the latter group was 2°C lower than the fat from the animals kept at the higher temperature. This means that fat from a cooler environment is liquid at relatively cool temperatures.

What does a melting point stand for? Heat is necessary to liquify solid fat. Thus an oil which is already liquid by nature must have inner warmth. In the above example this means that animals living in cold climates have to generate more heat within. Their fat therefore has a lower melting point. A lower melting point thus indicates more *inner* warmth. This is necessary so that in the cold climate their fats remain softer, do not harden, and the animals can move better.

It is significant in this regard that human fat has on average a much lower melting point than animal fats. This tells us that humans have far more inner warmth than animals. We are not speaking of body temperature but of warmth that has been interiorized and become substance.

In both human and animal, however, a distinction must be made between fat reserves or deposits and the fat in organs or protoplasm. The latter is a normal part of every cell. It is distributed in such a way that it is not visible. Fat deposits, on the other hand, are found above all in the fatty tissue layer under the skin and around some inner organs. Certain areas of the body are preferred, which contributes greatly to the shaping (or 'rounding') of the body. Deposit fat is a store of life, but does not get much involved in general metabolism; its melting point is relatively high. The fat in organs is highly active and has a lower melting point. (The 'hidden' fat present mainly in meat and eggs, which we are warned against nowadays, is an organ fat and therefore active.) We can see that the melting point of fats indicates their biological activity. This is also why milk fat (i.e. butter), which is an organ fat, cannot be considered the same as beef fat, which is deposit fat, although both come from the same animal.

From the above experiments and the occurrence of fats we can say that fat is primarily interiorized warmth—unlike carbohydrates, which are primarily condensed light. In other words, fat belongs by nature to the region above the earth where life forces have their origin, while carbohydrates come down to earth completely, and indeed partly 'turn to earth,' as in the formation of wood.

The activity of fats is connected with their interiorized warmth, which expresses itself in a low melting point. This has often led to a disastrous oversimplification: vegetable oils (liquid) = good, animal fats (solid) = bad. It is easy to see that this cannot be true, for coconut fat has a very high melting point, while whale oil, definitely of animal origin, has an extremely low melting point.

Chemists, of course, have long since investigated the basis of these differences in melting point. These are on the one hand the *length* of the fatty acid and on the other hand the degree of *saturation*. The longer—that is, the denser—a fatty acid, the higher its melting point. Saturation means that all possible bonds with the carbon elements are 'occupied,' that is, this fat cannot take up anything else, which gives the substance practically indefinite keeping qualities. It also means that our organism cannot so easily break it down and process it. Saturated fats always have higher melting points than unsaturated; they have solidified.

Unsaturated means that the fat has one or more 'double bonds.' These can still take up something else, and are thus more accessible to the organism's digestive juices. They can, however, also easily take up oxygen and go bad, that is, grow rancid. Then they have a bitter taste and are toxic.

The following example of four fatty acids of equal length that differ only in the number of double bonds can show how much a double bond changes the melting point.

Melting Point in Centigrade

stearic acid	+70°
oleic acid (one double bond)	+13°
linoleic acid (two double bonds)	-5°
linolenic acid (three double bonds	-11°

This drop in the melting point of oils which otherwise have the same chain length makes it immediately evident that the substance is inwardly warmed through and activated by the presence of double bonds. As a result, active fats are easily broken down and processed in the organism, which gives them their biological value. Originally these fatty acids were therefore referred to as vitamin F. Such 'openness' also means, however, that highly unsaturated fats are very easily changed by oxygen from the air, by heat and by light. This results in rancid, highly indigestible and even toxic products. These active oils should therefore never be used for frying. And when stored they must protected from light, air, and warmth.

This is why nature produces a saturated and hard fat in the tropics (palm oil and coconut fat): though they grow in warm temperatures, they cannot become rancid. But they are also difficult for the body to digest.

The idea of biological value has led again to a certain oversimplification: the more double bonds (i.e. the more unsaturated), the better. 'Rich in unsaturated fatty acids' means high quality nowadays. Unfortunately this is not the case, as it is too limited a view. The position and angle of the double bonds also plays a role. There is a fatty acid with three double bonds (like the highly active linolenic acid) which nevertheless has a very high melting point (+ 48° C) and is biologically inactive. One finds it in the inedible wood oil. Furthermore, saying 'rich in unsaturated fatty acids,' for instance in regard to margarine, does not tell us anything about the level of saturation of the fatty acids in the remaining part of the product. In judging the quality of a fat, it is more important where it comes from and how it is processed than how many unsaturated fatty acids it contains.

Another common term which is meant to guarantee quality is 'pure vegetable fat.' This is because butter was given such a bad name for decades, saying it was low in unsaturated and high in saturated fatty acids, and worse still that it contained cholesterol, which supposedly causes heart attacks and many other diseases.

How much of this is true?

Butter

The German saying 'Everything is in butter' means that everything is going well. In the past, people evidently felt that butter was something both harmonious and beneficial.

Butter is milk fat obtained by a special manufacturing process. It is not only fat. Legally, butter must contain more than 80% fat and less than 20% water. It is made from the cream obtained by centrifuging milk. The cream is whipped until it separates into butter (fat) and buttermilk (protein and water). Butter is clearly a milk fat, that is an organ fat, completely different in composition from deposit fat or even from organ fat from the animal's *meat*. Depending on the manufacturing method, distinction is made between:

1. *Sweet cream butter:* butter made from unsoured pasteurized cream.

2. *Cultured butter:* butter made from soured cream. Cream is soured using a lactic acid culture and then made into butter. The souring makes the typical butter taste stronger.

3. *Farmhouse butter:* butter also made from soured cream, but unpasteurized. Souring is due to the natural souring of milk in this case. The taste is usually much more intense and the butter keeps less well than the other types.

4. *Clarified butter:* butter that contains practically no water, since careful heating has evaporated it. Therefore clarified butter will keep much longer than butter and above all, is suitable for frying.

If we compare butter with other fats, we find that it is much more *varied* in its composition. So far 76 different fatty acids have been identified. No other edible fat or oil comes anywhere near this. (Many oils have no more than five different fatty acids.) The fatty acids are both short and long, saturated and non-saturated, with single, double, and even four or five double bonds.

What does such universality, such variety, signify? It is a typically human phenomenon, for animals are always specialized in some way, and plants even more so. On the other hand, universality is something which always is or at least should be present at the beginning of development. Every young child is universally gifted and will only develop special aptitudes later. Even animals are far more universal in their embryonic development than they are later. Nature has produced milk as a universal food to match this—as a food for the newborn.

As already stated, the effect of a food rests not only on its composition and sourcez but on how it is processed. Fats need to be emulsified in the intestine before they enter into the blood. In healthy people, about three or four hours after a rich meal this leads to some cloudiness in the blood serum, which will disappear again within a few hours. The degree and duration of the clouding depend on the nature of the fats eaten. Generally speaking, hard, saturated fats cause a greater degree of clouding than highly unsaturated fatty acids. The latter may even shorten the clouding. The fat clouding test (lipemia test) can be used to get a rough idea of the biological value of a fat (see table below). It becomes evident through this test that heating a fat greatly reduces its biological value—even if the fatty acid composition does not change.

The following table (page 101) shows that highly active oils such as wheat germ oil and flaxseed oil do indeed have the biological value which is attributed to them, but only in

99

their raw form. Unpasteurized raw farmhouse butter comes next in the scale. It is interesting to note that sunflower oil is affected by heating although it still retains a positive biological value, and that frying has a negative effect on any kind of fat.

This is not really a surprise, for the more sensitive a person or a substance, the more vulnerable. It also means that the more active the oil, the more careful one should be in using it. Flaxseed oil has always been known to be highly active. This is why it needs to be protected from light, air (oxygen) and heat, as these will alter it. Left exposed, it will harden and turn into varnish ('linseed oil').

Therefore, highly active oils should never be used for frying! Only universal fats, which also contain some saturated (stabile) fatty acids, are suitable. Among these are butter, clarified butter, olive oil, sunflower oil and sesame oil (widely used in Asia). They are suitable for frying food in small quantities of fat for no longer than ten minutes. These fats are not completely inactive, but robust enough. Frying calls for high temperatures. The higher the temperatures a fat will tolerate, the more suited it is to the purpose. Deep fat frying, that is, submerging food in large quantities of fat at high temperatures for a longer time, is always a problem. Inactive fats like coconut or peanut oil can be used for this purpose because they do not alter with high temperatures, and are in any case better than all other synthetically hardened frying fats on the market today. However, it should be borne in mind that the good frying qualities of these oils come at the cost of bad biological value. Coconut and peanut oil are at least of natural origin and not processed. It is technically very easy today to make completely hardened fats which are then sold as frying fat. One can expose these fats to the sun, one can even heat them to the highest temperatures and use them repeatedly (almost) without limit and they will not turn rancid. They are so saturated that they do not alter anymore. On the other hand, these fats are a burden on metabolism. This

Biological Rating of Different Oils and Fats
Based on Lipemia Test

	Points	Fat Tested	Processing	State
Positive Values	160	wheat germ oil	cold pressed, raw	raw
	157	flaxseed oil	cold pressed, raw	
	133	sunflower oil	cold pressed, raw	
	132	farmhouse butter	unpasteurized, raw	
	126	goose fat	raw	
	120	pork back fat	raw	
	100	butter	raw	
	81	health food margarine	raw	
	50	peanut oil	cold pressed, raw	
	28	ordinary margarine	raw	
Negative Values	20	sunflower oil	cold pressed, 110°C	heated
	6	chicken fat	100°C	
	2	health food margarine	100°C	
	1	butter	100°C	
	31	goose fat	100°C	
	52	pork fat	100°C	
	70	ordinary edible oil	100°C	
	73	ordinary margarine	100°C	
	74	butter	200°C	
	98	ordinary edible oil	200°C	
	98	ordinary margarine	200°C	
	107	sheep fat	100°C	
	111	beef fat	100°C	
	127	goose fat	200°C	fried
	140	pork fat	200°C	
	160	hardened vegetable fat	200°C	
	175	beef fat	200°C	
	188	sheep fat	200°C	

Bober H., *Medizin und Ernährung 3, 12* (1962), pp. 269-274

shows that frying presents problems whichever way you look at it. Healthy individuals do not, of course, have to do without it. But in earlier times people considered frying or roasting to be something for festive occasions, not for everyday use like nowadays.

It is the high temperatures used in roasting and frying that release the delightful aromas and flavors. This cannot be achieved at anything like this level by boiling, though grilling or toasting will also achieve it. However, we need to understand that frying and roasting put a strain on the liver and gall bladder system! Someone with normal health will cope well, providing it is done in moderation. In recent years, however, the consumption of fried and roasted products (for instance, coffee!) has increased more and more, and this has weakened the liver of more people than ever before.[14]

Margarine

From early times people always equated 'fat' with wealth and 'thin' or 'lean' with poverty. In hard periods such as wartime, a 'fat deficit' always arises. Napoleon III realized this, particularly its effect on conducting war, when he was preparing a preventive action against Prussia. A few weeks after the battle of Koeniggraetz (3 July, 1866), in which he had suffered a stunning defeat, he therefore gave order for a cheap fat to be developed that would be easy to transport and would keep well. A prize of 100,000 francs was announced (a vast sum in those days!). After many experiments, 'oleomargarine'was produced. It was marketed under such names as 'synthetic butter,' 'low-cost butter' and many others.

The name 'margarine' prevailed at a later time. The original margarine was 100% beef fat. Later, vegetable oils and above all whale oil, which was very cheap, were used to produce margarine. But these liquid oils first had to be hardened so that they could be spread on bread. A process of hardening fats was invented in which hydrogen is added to the unsaturated fats to 'saturate' them. This raises the melting point of the oils. Their taste is also lost, which was important in the case of whale oil. The road was now free for mass production of cheap fat. The decades which followed brought continuous improvements. 'Synthetic butter' became a product in its own right, which was no longer simply like butter, but in the eyes of many consumers even better, meaning higher quality and healthier. 'Well-informed' people who were careful to eat healthy food therefore chose margarine.

How did such a change come about? It was based on a single scientific study. Russian scientists fed rabbits on a diet containing butter and eggs for a length of time. The animals then showed massive deposits in their blood vessels, which were found to be cholesterol. Such deposits are also found in humans with arteriosclerosis. Over time the deposits calcify and lead to heart attacks. People thought they had now 'discovered' where these deposits come from—from butter and eggs. They thought they had finally found the cause not only of this typical ailment of old age, but also of many other diseases, above all the dreaded angina pectoris which may lead to heart attack. The consequence was a relentless search to identify cholesterol as the root cause of age-related changes as well as other ills.

An important fact was overlooked, however. The original experimental design was fundamentally flawed, for rabbits do not normally eat butter or eggs. Their organism is not designed for them! They simply *have* to get sick if forced to feed on a completely unnatural diet because this food is against their nature, just as humans would get sick if forced to eat grass. Since this was not considered, the conclusions of this experiment are invalid. In spite of this, warnings against cholesterol were issued; indeed, a whole propaganda campaign was launched. Since most people had never heard of cholesterol anyway, they were greatly reassured to be informed that a 'dangerous' substance that causes heart disease and other ailments is *not* present in a particular food. (See 'The Cholesterol Problem,' page 110, for a detailed discussion.)

Until about 150 years ago, general nutrition was undoubtedly low in fat. Most people at that time were poor and hungry. This resulted in specific diseases, above all tuberculosis, which always develops in places where nutrition is deficient in fat. Fats were always much more expensive than such foods as potatoes, bread and beans, the food of the poor. Fat is much more satisfying, however, as it has more than twice the calories of carbohydrates or proteins. Thus it was known that a basic treatment for tuberculosis was a diet high in fats. Rising prosperity meant that fat consumption rose enormously. This was a major factor in eliminating tuberculosis. In more recent decades, fats have become relatively cheap and the food of the 'affluent' is available to more or less the whole population. Therefore, more and more fat has been consumed, more than is good for people. Inevitably this has led to diseases which are the exact opposite of tuberculosis—fatty degeneration of organs, especially 'fatty liver' (a disease of affluence). The condition is widespread today, though it often goes unrecognized. (But the distinct increase in obesity, especially in Western countries, is not principally due to fat consumption. It is due to an excessive intake of 'empty' calories, especially sugar, but there are also other causes.)

Starting in the 1970s, overweight, fatty liver and fat deposits in blood vessels finally induced the medical profession to warn against animal fats, which on top of it also contain cholesterol. As always, simplified messages are highly suggestive. Fear of animal fats reached the level of panic. 'Low fat' thus became a mark of quality. To what extent is this justified?

It is a psychological phenomenon that people tend to go from one extreme that is seen as harmful to the other extreme, and fail to realize that both extremes are harmful. Once people knew that excessive fat consumption leads to illness, simple logic should have told them to limit the amount of fat in their diet. But this would have made their food much less interesting, since only dishes which have plenty of fat are tasty. Tastiness is equated with 'good.' This is why the demand arose not for a reduction in fats but for a product that would look like fat and could be used just like it, without being fat. The whole range of 'light' products benefited from this fear. They are 'low' in fat, sugar, nicotine, and so on.

Margarine manufacturers benefited greatly from the fear of animal fats. They were able to say that margarine is a pure vegetable product, cholesterol-free, high in unsaturated fatty acids, and so on, and therefore superior to butter.

What is the real situation? As already stated, it is not right to put all 'animal fats' in the same category. We have seen that milk fat, i.e. butter, has the characteristic of universality. It actually occupies the middle position among all fats. Its ability to be spread on bread—as compared to oils and tallow—also indicates that it is right in the middle, at the transition between liquid and solid.

This was just the problem that margarine manufacturers faced: how to achieve the semisolid state of spreadability. The solution was to harden fats with low melting points. Whales are almost extinct and protected, so that cheap whale oil was no longer available. This is why any margarine, even the cheapest, can be declared 'pure vegetable fat.' It is based primarily on rapeseed oil, grown especially in Europe. To this day, in Central Europe rape is grown almost entirely for margarine production and is even subsidized for that purpose! In the past, however, most people evidently did not find the taste of rapeseed oil appealing at all, which is why it was practically used only for technical purposes, for instance to oil machines. Later on, feeding experiments produced astonishing results. It was found that rapeseed oil fed to seven (!) different animal species caused *massive damage to the heart*. One would think that people would act in accord with such findings, but the only result was a suggestion to 'review' the use of rapeseed oil for human consumption.

Here we have not just a general psychological problem but also an economic one because of the legal status of subsidies for rapeseed oil, which is difficult to change. What should be done when something proves harmful? Rather than doing without the object in question, the harmful component is identified, and efforts are made to eliminate or limit it. This happens in the case of caffeine in coffee, tar in cigarettes—and erucic acid in rape oil. Rape contains up to 40% erucic acid, which was identified as being the problem. Rather than eliminate rape, people developed varieties low in erucic acid. Officially they still contain 1% or 2% of the erucic acid. With this kind of selective breeding, people forget that a plant is a whole. Intervention in one part will inevitably also have an effect on other qualities. Thus for instance, it is possible today to grow roses without the 'nuisance' of thorns, but the result is a rose that has no more scent. Breeding to get rid of the erucic acid does not mean that rape oil is the ideal fat. It is grotesque that margarine, made largely from rape oil, has been recommended by so-called scientists all over the world for the prevention of heart disease. Erucic acid is also found in peanuts, by the way, whose peculiarity was pointed out earlier. There are, of course, also margarines that consist only of sunflower oil according to the declaration on the package.

Oil has to be hardened to make it spreadable. The methods have been fully researched by now and brought to technical perfection. The double bonds which give unsaturated fatty acids their biological value are either 'saturated' (with hydrogen) or displaced (this is called 'partial hardening'). The melting point will in any case go up, but the biological value goes down! This will make the oil spreadable, that is, butter-like. Of course, it is possible to add in unprocessed oil that is still active (the margarine will then be labeled 'rich in unsaturated fats'), but this has to be made up for by hardening the other oils much more. Emulsifiers will also be needed to combine the two fats. So-called 'organic' margarines are made out of fats which are naturally hard, such as palm oil or coconut fat. The product can then be declared to be 'free of hardened fats.' (Palm oil and coconut fat are naturally hard, and therefore saturated.)

Because the fats in margarine have gone through extensive changes, their fat-soluble vitamins are largely destroyed. It is therefore a legal requirement to add vitamins A and D artificially, otherwise people would develop serious deficiencies. In Germany, the law also requires that some starch be added to margarine so that any admixture of butter, which is not permitted, may be more easily detected.

Knowing the chemistry of fats, it is possible to vary them and produce fats that will exactly meet consumers' wishes. The question of what happens to biological values is here completely ignored. Highly saturated fats specially tailored to the baking trade, for instance, are called 'shortenings.' They seem not to be hard because 10% to 15% nitrogen is incorporated, which makes them appear light and creamy. All these industrially processed and highly specialized fats are produced to meet the wishes of consumers (bakers, chefs, domestic cooks) who are only interested in the properties for the baking and appearance of the finished product—and these are simply outstanding! Who will ask about biological value if the fat is so easy to use and has reliable properties? People do not even notice that the taste has suffered too in this process of 'perfection.'

The ultimate development in the area of fats is 'fat-free fat.' As already mentioned, the 'nutritional value' of fat is much higher than that of carbohydrates or protein. The conclusion has been that fat makes a person fat. This is not untrue, but it only applies within limits. In the metabolism, the organism is able to deal freely with the three substances of life—carbohydrates, proteins and fats—and can even make fat out of sugar. Actually, fat does not make one fat, since its satiating effect is long-lasting. Sugar, in contrast, makes one very hungry after a short time because the initial rapid increase of sugar in the blood is followed by a rapid decrease to subnormal levels, giving rise to hunger pangs.

People are also still unjustifiably afraid of cholesterol. As a lipoid it is 'fat-like' and also found in 'hidden' fats. The obvious conclusion for those afraid of fats would be, as mentioned before, to limit their fat consumption, but that means a sacrifice. Of course, no one wants to do this because then the flavor is lost. Therefore 'light' products are made available—'as-if' products that pretend to be something they really are not.

This continues the trend established with caffeine-free coffee, sugar-free sweets, creamless coffee creamer, meat-free (soy) frankfurters and meatballs, and so on. They offer consumers an almost perfect illusion, allowing them to sin without regret. This takes away the bad conscience people have when consuming them. A German trade mark for low-fat products is 'You may!'

This is why fat-free fat was invented in the United States. The contradictory name means that chemically the substance is a fat, but the organism does not recognize it as such. Therefore it cannot be broken down in the metabolism, nor is it taken up into the organism. It is eliminated unchanged with the feces. Like practically all hardened fats, this 'fat' is completely tasteless. It does, however, create the typical feeling in the mouth that one gets from fats. Meals gain that 'rounded' taste that people like and simply do not want to do without.

Technically *olestra*, which is the official name of fat-free fat, is produced by linking sugar with eight fatty acids. The manufacturers, the American firm Procter & Gamble, took out a patent on it as early as 1971. It took 25 years of discussion, however, with 125,000 pages of expert opinions, before permission was obtained to sell olestra under the trade name 'Olean.' So far it is used only in potato chips and other snack foods, which are (usually) only eaten in limited amounts. It has since been found that the product may cause diarrhea (as one would have expected). It also inhibits the absorption of fat-soluble vitamins such as A, D, E and K. In spite of this, the worldwide triumphal march of the product will no doubt continue. It did, after all, cost some 200 million dollars to develop this cheap fat-free fat.

The Cholesterol Problem

What is cholesterol? It was described as early as the 18th century as a 'fatty wax.' Later, it was found in gallstones (the name *cholesterol* means 'hard bile' in Greek). It is a fat-*like* substance (a lip*oid*). Investigation has shown it to be present in the membrane of every cell in the body. It serves the delimiting function of the cell membrane and is essential for substance transfer through the membrane, where it has a mediating function. Cholesterol is thus a substance which is necessary for life, above all as a vehicle for constructive metabolic processes. This is why it is found especially in egg yolk, from which the future embryo will develop. It is also present—in much smaller amounts—in milk, which serves to supply infants with life forces. It is the same with butter. In humans, high cholesterol levels are found in the outer layer of the adrenal gland, which is likewise a mediator of constructive impulses.

Cholesterol is the parent substance for many highly important substances needed for life. Examples are the bile acids, the male and female hormones, the cortisone which the body produces itself, and provitamin D. The organism would not be able to produce any of these without cholesterol! To repeat: Cholesterol is a substance which is essential for life. Later generations will find it a psychological enigma how it was possible to give cholesterol such a bad name in our time. For some time now scientists have begun to recognize that cholesterol is not so bad after all.[15]

Factually, it is of course correct that elevated cholesterol levels are pathological and may lead to arteriosclerosis. But first of all the question is: what is an increased level of cholesterol in the blood? This is a controversial issue among doctors. The normal level of cholesterol used to be under 300 mg/dl (7.8 mmol/1) because most healthy people have levels between 250 and 300 mg/dl. In recent decades the 'normal level' has been continually reduced down to today's 200 mg/dl (5.2 mmol/1), which is usually only achievable through taking medicine. In any case, over 300 mg/dl is clearly too high and pathological. Then again, a high level of *any* substance is pathological! Raised blood sugar levels are just as pathological, as are raised uric acid levels. The question is, how do such raised levels come about at all?

With cholesterol, the 'guilty party' was soon found: food. People failed to realize that the above-mentioned 'fundamental' experiments on rabbits (see page 103) were based on completely false premises. Thus we have here the same evident (yet unnoticed) error as in the case of BSE, mad 'cow' disease (see page 14). Yet for years cholesterol in food was said to be responsible for deposits in the arteries and the diseases they caused, heart attacks being only one example. No one took note of the fact that the body *itself* produces cholesterol. Its levels are difficult to determine; they can really only be estimated. Different figures are given by different authors. Production is about 5 to 8 *grams* a day, with a total amount in the whole organism of about 200 grams. 100 grams of butter contain about 280 *milli*grams of cholesterol. This is therefore hardly of any significance whatsoever, even if butter consumption is high (meat has higher cholesterol levels than butter, although still in milligrams). In spite of this it has been possible to make people all over the world consider butter (not meat!) to be dangerous, recommending margarine instead. One egg contains just over 280 milligrams of cholesterol on average. Even three eggs will not yet amount to 1 gram of cholesterol, which is a great deal less than the amount produced by our own organism. Instead of realizing that the body itself produces much greater quantities of cholesterol than can ever be taken in through food, science gets lost in secondary details like LDL cholesterol and HDL cholesterol.

It is nevertheless right to say that in these prosperous times, consumption of fat, meat and eggs is well above the acceptable level.

It has also been discovered that the diseases for which cholesterol is held responsible are not caused by cholesterol itself, but rather by its *aging products*. These arise when cholesterol ages due to being heated to high temperatures or comes in contact with light or air (oxygen) through improper storage. Cholesterol is an active substance, as it has one of the double bonds referred to in the discussion of fats. This means it can take up substances and can also easily be broken down; it just cannot be inert. If it is nevertheless deposited in the blood vessels there must be other reasons. Only in recent years has it been possible technically to distinguish the aging products of cholesterol. It was found that the oxidation products of cholesterol are extremely dangerous. More than 80 of these have been found. Eating even the smallest amounts of them can lead to very serious changes in the blood vessels within 24 hours. Pure and fresh cholesterol, on the other hand, causes no problems at all because it can be broken down and metabolized. It is therefore quite possible that the deposited cholesterol does come from food, but it is food that is no longer fresh. It is the aging products of cholesterol which are dangerous. Such aging products had not been taken into account before. It appears, therefore, that it is not the intake of cholesterol itself which is the problem but its treatment, or rather maltreatment. The situation is similar to those described for milk and for bread baking. A fresh egg, fresh milk and fresh butter would be no problem with regard to their cholesterol content. But dried egg (in long lasting baked goods), dried milk, or butter that has been stored in the wrong way or heated to high temperatures would be another matter.

Above all, it is the way food is manipulated that decides the issue! It is known that the Maasai in Africa, who live almost entirely on milk, milk products and meat, and the Eskimos, who eat only animal fat and meat, do not have raised cholesterol levels, nor the diseases these may cause. It has to be considered, however, that these people only eat these foods fresh.

The real problem is thus not the intake of fresh fats but either the eating of maltreated fat or insufficient degradation of the body's self-produced cholesterol. In this latter case one can say if a substance which in itself is active is not being used, it becomes subject to other laws, such as gravity, which means deposition. This general law was expressed by Goethe in the words of his dramatic character, Faust:

> *What you have as inheritance,*
> *Earn it! Make it your own!*
> *What is not used, is a burden.*
> *Only what the moment makes—this we can use.*
>
> Faust I, Night

This also applies, for instance, to sugar. If the organism is unable to make use of it (as in diabetes) it will be eliminated, being soluble in blood. With cholesterol the situation is that if it is not used, it falls out of the blood, and being insoluble, is deposited in the blood vessels. This leads to arteriosclerosis, a typical disease of old age. If on the other hand the cholesterol is truly 'made one's own,' meaning further metabolized, the above-mentioned products are created: bile acids, sexual hormones, provitamin D, and self-produced cortisone. All of these become less in old age. A major factor in this decrease is insufficient cholesterol *degradation*. Thus, the high cholesterol levels in the blood and the forming of deposits are not the actual disease; they are the consequence of insufficient cholesterol degradation.

When it comes to food, therefore, it is better to give more consideration to the way a food has been treated or mistreated, than to the quantities of fats or saturated fatty acids and so on it contains. Fresh products which are still active can be taken hold of by the organism. Of course this calls for inner activity in the body. Such activity will then break down cholesterol.

It is known that activity keeps us young and healthy. Physical activity also helps to break down cholesterol through the warming effect of increased metabolism. However, it is important to consider *what kind* of activity we are talking about. The archetypal harmonious movement of human beings is walking; right into old age it creates balance, contributing to health and to vitality. An hour's walk a day (not a jog), for instance, contributes immensely to overall strength. For young people strong physical activity also is beneficial, while in older people *exaggerated* physical activity tends to lead to rigidity of the soul. Everything has its proper time. For older people it is *spiritual* activity which produces this mild form of breaking down that allows new building up to follow. We have considered this in detail in the discussion of lactic acid. It also holds true for cholesterol. Older people who are active in spirit and soul (not merely physically) stay 'young.' An ideal working together of bodily and spiritual activity can also be found in the movement art of eurythmy developed by Rudolf Steiner. In suitable form it is appropriate for any age.

One problem concerning fat which people are quite aware of, without knowing how to deal with it, is *obesity*. Up to 1980, every fourth person in the USA was said to be obese. Today it is every third, with the trend rising! No wonder that lay people have begun to think that fat is what makes one fat. A panic-level fear has developed of all natural fats, and people think the solution lies in 'light' products like margarine or fat-free fat—the very fats that have been mistreated. In reality, however, obesity is not a question of fat consumption alone. As already mentioned, the organism can easily convert protein and above all simple carbohydrates such as sugar into fat. The pancreas produces increased amounts of insulin when the blood sugar rises. Sugar is then converted not only to glycogen, the storage substance of the liver, but also to fat. At the same time fat is prevented from dissolving. The fat production is therefore triggered by the sudden rise in blood sugar which comes from indulging in sweets. Fat on its own need not cause obesity. Eskimos, who live on practically nothing but fat and protein, are not fat.

Eating too much of any food can doubtless cause obesity, but not in everyone. Simple observation will show that some people eat extremely little and yet fail to lose weight. Others again may eat large amounts and do not gain weight. Body weight is not simply a question of how many calories one eats. It has far more to do with the way one deals with the food one eats, that is, how one metabolizes.

Rudolf Steiner pointed out that human beings take nourishment not only from food. We can also receive life forces through the senses. This is understandable when considering what was said at the beginning. It is not so much the substances as such which are important, but the life they contain, and this ultimately comes from light. The extent to which these influences complement one another depends on the individual constitution. One person will be constitutionally 'round' and 'well padded,' another thin and gaunt.

With obesity the situation becomes pathological. Today people frequently eat sweets, pastries, chocolate, ice cream and so on. And usually it is not just a matter of 'empty' calories, such as sugar, but also the extremely hardened fats which these products contain. These are like 'stones' to the metabolism— difficult to get at. Thus the organism is not able to process them properly and has to place them in its fat deposits, or in the blood vessels.

Psychological factors play into this too, as has been known for a long time. The German expression *Kummerfett* ('worry fat') recognizes that eating can be a substitute for some other dissatisfaction. Eating sweets is not done just to satisfy hunger anyway. People can even be hungry but not satisfy it with a proper meal, possibly because they are afraid of fat and therefore go for food with sugar. Most people would find their way back to their natural constitution if they ate wholesome meals rather than 'junk food' consisting largely of empty calories that cannot really satisfy hunger. This has led to the paradoxical situation that most overweight people, above all young people, are found today among the *poorer* population.

In industrialized countries, *anorexia* soon followed on the heels of obesity. This refusal to eat is again a psychological problem. Both disorders can only be understood if we gain real insight into how human beings relate to their bodies. This is why, for instance, medical treatment alone will mostly have no effect. As mentioned before, food helps human beings to come to earth in the right way. Ultimately it is a spiritual problem. It concerns the relationship human beings have to the earth. Food is the means to this end. It will be necessary in the future to gain real insight into these matters and make fundamental changes. This will involve not only a different attitude to life in general and to education, but also a different attitude to nutrition.

Future Prospects

There can be no doubt that the average human life span has risen in recent years. This is usually presented, with conviction, as one of the achievements of modern medicine. But what is not mentioned is that most of the diseases that people used to die from had already decreased considerably long *before* modern drugs and vaccines existed. It is also a fact that people who are getting older today have many more health problems requiring constant treatment than earlier. In addition, more young people and children today are often ill, and chronically so. This means that the general constitution of humanity is getting weaker—and this is largely a problem of nutrition. For the future it will be necessary to gain clear insight into these matters. *Longer* life, or even *saving* life, is not the same as stronger health. The latter depends to a large extent on nutrition.

Fundamental insight into the nature of substances is also needed. From today's materialistic point of view, food is judged according to energy content and substances that can be measured. This is not wrong, but it is one-sided. The main point is the life which is in food. Life is a force and cannot be measured using only physical or chemical methods. A typical sign of the modern way of thinking is the often quoted pronouncement of philosopher L. Feuerbach: 'Man is what he eats.' (In German, *Der Mensch ist, was er isst!*) It is a play on the words *ist* ('is') and *isst* ('eats'). This is utter materialism. If it were true, someone who eats a lot of chicken would gradually turn into a chicken. The organism is protected from this by its digestive function (see page 51), which keeps foreign characteristics away. What is true in this statement is that if people do not eat the right food they will not be able to realize their life's meaning.

To overcome the materialistic way of thinking, it is also important to *cultivate the way we eat* our meals. This was done in the past. Many people today think eating is a waste of time. They simply do not have have that time, so a quick snack in between other things will do, possibly in front of the computer. The least effect of this will be to dull their sense of taste, but quite apart from that, they do not stop to reflect that they are dealing with a gift from God. People used to pray before meals and again afterwards to give thanks, yet today the inner attitude of thankfulness has largely been replaced by one of demanding.

As Angelus Silesius expressed it in the verse quoted at the beginning, what feeds us is not the bread but God's light and spirit, meaning that substance is in reality the bearer of forces. Today we can say that it is just as necessary to realize which force resides in which substance. This is addressed in another verse, attributed to Angelus Silesius as well. It is only seemingly in contradiction with the first verse (page 6), but in reality takes it further.

> *The bread feeds us indeed,*
> *if rightly we receive it.*
> *Through it we can reach*
> *Even to heaven itself.*

The message of those few words is that nutrition is not only a biological but also a spiritual matter. This we must know today. Of course we cannot 'eat our way to heaven,' but serious illness can be helped to heal through nutrition. And good nutrition is essential to maintain our health. Kollath, the nutritionist who because of his farsightedness was not always popular nor really understood, once said, rather sarcastically: 'Most people commit suicide with knife and fork.' This means that in these prosperous times many people make themselves ill with the food they eat, sometimes with fatal consequences.

The conclusion we draw from this should not be 'back to nature.' In the past, people had a direct relationship with the natural world. This has now been lost. Today we need to understand what the forces of life are and how to use them to support spiritual development.

We should certainly not discard the advances made in technology. But we need to understand that technology has developed from physics, a science concerned with dead substance. This is why in essence it destroys life. Thus the important thing is to use it with clear insight and only where compromises are necessary. In principle, Kollath's statement that foods should be as natural as possible holds true. But it should be emphasized once again that it is possible to take natural processes further by suitable methods. This has been shown by the example of lactic acid fermentation.

To carry this out, it will be necessary to let go of some agreeable habits which are not only unnecessary, but in the long run even harmful. Examples have been given here. Eating only food which gives pleasure all the time, and not just on festive occasions, leads not only to psychological changes but also to biological changes in the organism. It is important to understand today that the effects of nutrition are not superficial. They go much deeper than is generally acknowledged today.

References

GA = *volume number in the collected works of Rudolf Steiner in German*

1. Steiner R. *Health and Illness*, vol. 2 [GA 348]. New York: Anthroposophic Press, 1981 and 1983.

2. Husemann F./Wolff O. *The Anthroposophic Approach to Medicine*, vol. 3. Spring Valley, New York: Mercury Press, 2003.

3. Pottenger F. *Pottenger's Cats*. La Mesa, California: Price- Pottenger Foundation, 1983.

4. Kollath W. *Der Vollwert der Nahrung* [The Full Value of Food]. vols 1 and 2. Stuttgart: Wissenschaftliche Verlagsgesellschaft 1950, 1960.

5. Schoeneck A. *Sauer macht lustig!* [Sour cheers you up]. Stuttgart: Verlag Freies Geistesleben, 1990.

6. Wolff O. *Das Rätsel der Allergie* [The Riddle of Allergy]. Merkblatt No. 134, Berlin: Verein für Anthroposophisches Heilwesen.

7. Steiger D. Möglichkeiten und Grenzen zur Erfassung der ernährungs-physiologischen Qualität. [Possibilities and limits in determinating nutrition-physiological quality]. In Meyer-Ploeger und Vogtmann *Lebensmittelqualität* [Food Quality]. Karlsruhe 1991. Also *Merkurstab* 1993, p. 249.

8. Wolff O. *Zucker – Die süsse Sucht* [The Sweet Addiction]. Merkblatt Nr. 151. Berlin: Verein für Anthroposophisches Heilwesen.

9. Feingold B. *Why your Child is Hyperactive*. New York: Random House, 1974.

10. Hafer H. *Die heimliche Droge Nahrungsphosphat*. Heidelberg: Verlag Huethig, 1998. Published in English as *The Hidden Drug: Dietary Phosphate*. Phosadd, Australia: Armadale, 2001.

11. Wolff O. The hyperkinetic syndrome. *Journal of Anthroposophic Medicine*. 1993, Vol. 10, No. 3, p. 7-15.

12. Wolff O. *Home Remedies*. Edinburgh: Floris Books, 2000.

13. Grohmann, G. *The Plant*. Great Barrington: SteinerBooks, 1989.

14. Wolff O. *Die Leber - Organ der Lebenskraft* [The Liver – Organ of Vital Strength], Merkblatt Nr. 49. Berlin: Verein für Anthroposophisches Heilwesen.

15. Hartenbach W. *Die Cholesterin-Lüge* [The Cholesterol Lie]. München: Herbig Verlag, 2009; see also: Columbani P. *Fette Irrtümer:Ernährungsmythen Entlarvt* [Fat Errors: Food Myths Unmasked]. Zürich: Orell Füssli Verlag, 2010

liked her writing on Journaling, which is so important
and also Memories. Many women do not want to believe
abuse happened to them and some spend a lifetime running from the pain. I love that Cora brought scripture,
essential oils and prayer into every chapter. I have been
with Cora for a few sessions of massage therapy and was
very blessed. She always prayed before we started. I
would encourage you to check out her book and have
the courage to start your healing journey with Jesus and
Cora will be there also to answer any questions or pray
for you! You are loved!

—**Charlene Hanson,** Author and Director *of Women*
Courage

***

Blalack is raw, vulnerable, and candid. In her ground
breaking, introductory healing handbook Blalack tackle
the all-too-common problem of sexual assault and fan
ily trauma. Uncovering the deep wounds so many of
and our loved ones live with, that so many people co
tinuously want to ignore.

Real talk is authentically and creatively interwoven w
God's Word in this useful and deep-diving handbo
which includes hands-on healing guidelines, therapeu
uses for essential oils, and breathing exercises.

—**Kara L. Simpson**, CMT, RYT-200, Bodywork
structor & Owner of Humboldt Healing Arts

REVIEWS FC

MOVING FROM VIOLATED TO V

Essential oils have been known since Bibli
fact, to quote Dr. Axe, "at least 33 specific e
and aromatic oil producing plants are mentio
Bible, and the word 'incense' is mentioned 68
Scripture. Psalm 45:7-8, Proverbs 27:9, Isa. (
Hebrews 1:9 all reference oils in some way as in
of joy' and 'the oil of gladness,' and they speak o
oils 'rejoice the heart.' "

Chronicling her journey from abuse to faith, C
Blalack shares how essential oils mentioned in Goo
Word have played a major role in her emotional healing
incorporating objective Scriptural truth as the basis for
her new life in the Lord Jesus Christ. Her work is a
powerful testimony to God's transforming power
through His love, mercy, forgiveness and grace.
—**David R. Nicholas**, M.S., Th.D. President, *Shasta
Bible College & Graduate School*

***

I have known Cora since she was young, and have been
blessed to see the woman of God she has become, plus
a wonderful wife and mom! You will be so blessed, challenged, and find healing as you read her story and hear
her heart.

Moving from Violated to Victory

A Sexual Trauma Survivors Somatic Series

CORAJEAN BLALACK

Published by KHARIS PUBLISHING, an imprint of KHARIS MEDIA LLC.

Copyright © 2020 Corajean Blalack

ISBN-13: 978-1-946277-73-2

ISBN-10: 1-946277-73-8

Library of Congress Control Number: 2020943680

All rights reserved worldwide. All KHARIS PUBLISHING products are available at special quantity discounts for bulk purchase for sales promotions, premiums, fund-raising, and educational needs. For details, contact:

Kharis Media LLC
Tel: 1-479-599-8657
support@kharispublishing.com
www.kharispublishing.com

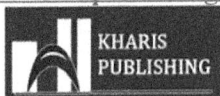

KHARIS
PUBLISHING

CONTENTS

	Introduction	vii
1	Memories	1
2	Dunamis	8
3	Rejection	20
4	Pleasure	35
5	Belly	46
6	Heart	57
7	Faith Healing? Yes Please!	65

Part 2

8	The Sequences	77
9	Session 1	93
10	Session 2	104
11	Session 3	109
	Final Thoughts and Farewell	116

INTRODUCTION

Between Us

> *May The Lord answer you when you are in distress; may The Name of The God of Jacob protect you.* Psalm 20:1

Suggested Oils:

Tea Tree - The oil of energetic boundaries

> *Cleanser by nature, tea tree oil clears negative energetic baggage. It specifically releases co-dependent and parasitic relationships. Tea Tree encourages individuals to relinquish all forms of self-betrayal.*

Frankincense - The oil of Truth

> *Frankincense reveals deceptions and false truths. This oil helps create new perspectives based on light and truth.*[1]

Greetings and Salutations. My name is Cora. I am qualified to speak to you on this topic because I have come through the misery, humiliation, shame, and training of long-term childhood sexual abuse—not just a survivor, but a total thriver. This is by following God. Believing God is who He says He is. Knowing Him. Loving Him.

In this work, I endeavor to lead a fellow survivor through some training God gave me by focusing on hot spots like memories, fear, and pleasure. The objective of this book is

---

[1] All the essential oil emotional definitions are taken directly out of the book 'Essential Emotions: Your Guide to Process, Release, and Live Free. 8th Edition'

to reach the ravaged soul—wherever she may be—and to show her how to believe and use God's Word, talk to God, and apply essential oils and loving touch to allow God (for He waits for us to accept Him) to bring her into wholeness.

God's Word is powerful and effective in healing our spirits, souls, hearts, and minds; even our bodies. Jesus, at times of certain healing, used His own spit, or mud, or water from the river. In other words, even Jesus used physical substance to accompany His Word. Sexual abuse trains our bodies, not just our minds. Using oils and massage to dissolve the hurtful touch and retrain the body to respond appropriately to loving touch is a 'physical substance' step we all need to take to complete healing. Most of us anyways.

This book is for any female who has been touched outside the safety of loving, holy wedlock. It was written with the traumatized in mind, for those who may be experiencing life dominating thought patterns and habits as a result of the violation of sexual abuse. We know that sex is dynamite; it must needs be handled properly to work like we want it to. Those parameters are set forth for us in God's Word. He knows how we ought to handle sex because He invented it.

Our bodies are temples of God. Our sexual unions, within the boundaries of holy matrimony, are designed by God to be living pictures of the relationship Christ wants to have with His church. Paul says this is a deep mystery. Sex becomes a type of sacred worship a married couple offers to God and sex outside of that picture is sin according to His Word. Therefore, it is harmful to our person. Let us stop taking our cues from the fickle and fake world on how to handle our sex lives and begin to listen to and follow The Ancient of Days, The One who truly knows how to guide us into honest, lasting, satisfying and glorious sexy sex.

This book is written from the perspective of a girl who achieved wholeness by following The Almighty, as described in the Christian Bible. Matthew 5:45 states *so that you may be sons of your Father who is in heaven. For he makes His sun on the evil and on the good, and sends rain on the just and on the unjust.* It is my firm and complete conviction that it is Jesus, and none other, who heals us. Yet, there are others who have different convictions and beliefs. I respect and honor that. Jesus is the Author of freewill. He tells us God spreads broadcast, good things like rain and sunshine, be you a believer or not. I don't personally believe whole healing is possible apart from one's relationship with The Living God. However, I do know that positive thought, intentions, and different healing activities can sometimes carry immeasurable power to transform us. Do not allow a difference in faith to stop you from using this book to pursue wholeness. I have practiced these massage sequences on ladies who didn't have the same convictions as I, and they were helped.

For over twenty years I have been asking God, *How can I achieve a level of healing fast, and bypass all the destruction this perverted training wants to execute in my life?*

I think the answer is here. Renew the mind. Recover the heart. Retrain the gut. Apply healing touch to affected areas. Over and through all this is the eternal pleasure and blessing of walking with The One who is Faithful and True.

I'm interested in hearing from you. [cora@gutsandvictory.com] I would be so thrilled to hear your story and speak blessing over you. My hope is that you are finding your own way to victory and a lifestyle that testifies of thriving through Him!

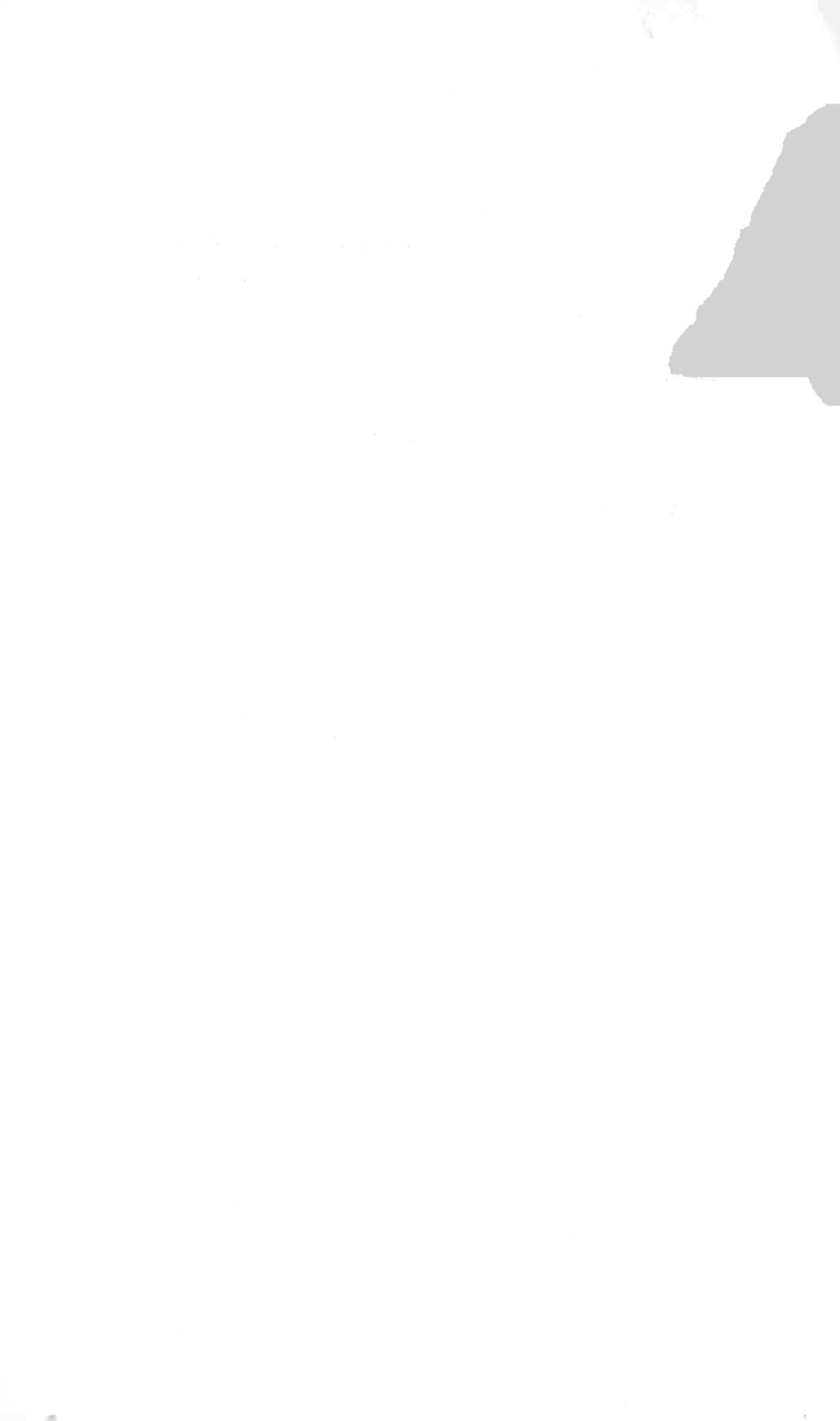

I liked her writing on Journaling, which is so important and also Memories. Many women do not want to believe abuse happened to them and some spend a lifetime running from the pain. I love that Cora brought scripture, essential oils and prayer into every chapter. I have been with Cora for a few sessions of massage therapy and was very blessed. She always prayed before we started. I would encourage you to check out her book and have the courage to start your healing journey with Jesus and Cora will be there also to answer any questions or pray for you! You are loved!

—**Charlene Hanson,** Author and Director *of Women of Courage*

***

Blalack is raw, vulnerable, and candid. In her groundbreaking, introductory healing handbook Blalack tackles the all-too-common problem of sexual assault and family trauma. Uncovering the deep wounds so many of us and our loved ones live with, that so many people continuously want to ignore.

Real talk is authentically and creatively interwoven with God's Word in this useful and deep-diving handbook which includes hands-on healing guidelines, therapeutic uses for essential oils, and breathing exercises.

—**Kara L. Simpson**, CMT, RYT-200, Bodywork Instructor & Owner of Humboldt Healing Arts

REVIEWS FOR

MOVING FROM VIOLATED TO VICTORY

Essential oils have been known since Biblical times. In fact, to quote Dr. Axe, "at least 33 specific essential oils and aromatic oil producing plants are mentioned in the Bible, and the word 'incense' is mentioned 68 times in Scripture. Psalm 45:7-8, Proverbs 27:9, Isa. 63:1 and Hebrews 1:9 all reference oils in some way as in 'the oil of joy' and 'the oil of gladness,' and they speak of how oils 'rejoice the heart.' "

Chronicling her journey from abuse to faith, Cora Blalack shares how essential oils mentioned in God's Word have played a major role in her emotional healing; incorporating objective Scriptural truth as the basis for her new life in the Lord Jesus Christ. Her work is a powerful testimony to God's transforming power through His love, mercy, forgiveness and grace.

—David R. Nicholas, M.S., Th.D. President, *Shasta Bible College & Graduate School*

***

I have known Cora since she was young, and have been blessed to see the woman of God she has become, plus a wonderful wife and mom! You will be so blessed, challenged, and find healing as you read her story and hear her heart.

This book is written from the perspective of a girl who achieved wholeness by following The Almighty, as described in the Christian Bible. Matthew 5:45 states *so that you may be sons of your Father who is in heaven. For he makes His sun rise on the evil and on the good, and sends rain on the just and on the unjust.* It is my firm and complete conviction that it is Jesus, and none other, who heals us. Yet, there are others who have different convictions and beliefs. I respect and honor that. Jesus is the Author of freewill. He tells us God spreads broadcast, good things like rain and sunshine, be you a believer or not. I don't personally believe whole healing is possible apart from one's relationship with The Living God. However, I do know that positive thought, intentions, and different healing activities can sometimes carry immeasurable power to transform us. Do not allow a difference in faith to stop you from using this book to pursue wholeness. I have practiced these massage sequences on ladies who didn't have the same convictions as I, and they were helped.

For over twenty years I have been asking God, *How can I achieve a level of healing fast, and bypass all the destruction this perverted training wants to execute in my life?*

I think the answer is here. Renew the mind. Recover the heart. Retrain the gut. Apply healing touch to affected areas. Over and through all this is the eternal pleasure and blessing of walking with The One who is Faithful and True.

I'm interested in hearing from you. [cora@gutsandvictory.com] I would be so thrilled to hear your story and speak blessing over you. My hope is that you are finding your own way to victory and a lifestyle that testifies of thriving through Him!

CHAPTER ONE

Memories

*M*ay He send you help from the sanctuary and grant
you support from Zion.
Psalm 20:2

Suggested Oils:

Black Pepper - The oil of unmasking

"Black Pepper reveals the masks and facades used to hide aspects of the self. Black Pepper also reignites the soul fire, fueling motivation and high energy, and hastening the healing process."

Ylang Ylang - The oil of the inner child

"Ylang Ylang reconnects individuals with the inner child and the pure, simple ways of the heart. This oil allows emotional healing to flow naturally, nurturing the heart through the process."

1

Memories

A cloudy cuppa joe.

There is much confusion that surrounds recovering memories of sexual abuse. Nobody wants to believe it's actually happening—much less to themselves or anyone they know. Because we don't want to believe it, what do we do? A myriad of reactions for sure. One thing we do, is doubt ourselves. This doubt is a messenger who heralds in confusion clouding the pictures in our minds that want to show us what is past. Occurrences that are, at the very least, uncomfortable. Pictures of memories that, when voiced, make those around us, who are often the perpetrator or intimately acquainted with the perpetrator, desperate to find an explanation that explains away this unthinkable, most destructive, vision. And we agree.

Let's work together for plausible deniability.

We are people. We lie. It's something we're good at. Every single person on the face of the earth is somehow, somewhere, in some way resting in the comfort of a covering up of the truth. A lie. A fib. A falsehood. A skirting around the truth. Some denial, or a simple omission. My spiritual mother has said, "If we could see ourselves as we really are, we'd run screaming into the night." Probably none of us are prepared for a full disclosure on the subject of ourselves. That's okay. It's a journey. One step. Then another. And so on.

We're liars searching for a truth we don't want because we somehow understand exposing the truth is the only way to move forward and be free.

2 Corinthians 3:17

> *Now The Lord is The Spirit; and where The Spirit of The Lord is, there is liberty.*

If I can't trust myself, and I don't, then I won't be capable of trusting. And because I can't trust myself to identify another who is trustworthy, I'm sunk.

Some of us are okay with being sunk. We resign ourselves to the hand we're dealt and accept it as our identity and reality. We're moving headlong into a chaotic life that keeps us on a spin cycle of roller-coasting between being okay—like maybe living a dream is possible—back to 'how did I get mixed up in this' trauma-creating situation; and then start the cycle again.

There do exist those brave souls that refuse. "No thanks," they say. I believe. I believe. I believe. I believe there is freedom to be had. And maybe this person has no idea how to reach it. Still, they reject identifying with and holding onto a trauma-inspired world view. It is to those daring hearts I speak.

Well, spit it out already.

I may only offer what I know to be true for myself, the path that worked for me. I do believe—am completely and utterly convinced—that this path has the power to work for every individual that dares step upon it. Because the map is alive!

Hebrews 4:12

> *For The Word of God is living and active and sharper than any two-edged sword, and piercing as far as the division of soul and spirit, of both joints and marrow, and able to judge the thoughts and intentions of the heart.*

It may therefore speak and guide, not to a category of symptoms, to the general, generic abused hordes. No, it has power to reach in and access the deepest most intimate fathoms of the singular, unique, one and only you.

I know because it happened to me. It's God's Word, bae-bae, believe it or not.

John 8:31-32

> *Then Jesus said to those Jews who believed Him, "If you abide in my Word you are my disciples indeed. And you shall know the Truth, and the Truth shall set you free."*

What does this have to do with my memories, my story, my issues, and desires? If we will choose to believe Jesus, he says we can abide, dwell, live, linger, rest, stay in His Word and know the Truth.

My guts heave and a sigh of relief issues forth from my lungs when I internalize the reality that I can know the real Truth. Thank you, Jesus! I praise You for the Truth.

And that Truth will free us. He is talking about the Truth of His Word. This applies to the individual's ability to remember rightly one's own memories, or truthfully see the self. Let's dig in.

Psalms 51:5-12

> *Behold, I was brought forth in iniquity, and in sin my mother conceived me. Behold, you desire truth in the inward parts, and in the hidden part you will make me to know wisdom. Purge me with hyssop and I shall be clean; wash me and I shall be whiter than snow. Make me hear joy and gladness, that the bones you have broken may rejoice. Hide your face from my sins and blot out all my iniquities.*

Create in me a clean heart, oh God, and renew a steadfast spirit within me. Do not cast me away from your Presence and do not take Your Holy Spirit from me. Restore to me the joy of your salvation and uphold me by your Righteous Spirit.

Our God wants us to have Truth in us. If we've hidden, and buried deep within ourselves situations that we absolutely were not equipped to handle (no one is equipped) and were not protected from, in an attempt to protect ourselves, we set up a stronghold against truth. It's okay; it's not a fault or blame. It's one miraculous way we are created. It's normal. The problem is if we leave it in the darkness, it will begin to operate on its own. It must be brought to light. The Light of Jesus. We know we need to honestly recover some parts of our memories. The memories are there already. Jesus will give us peace to be able to relax and have confidence that when they surface, they are indeed true. He is our Assurance. His Holy Spirit, The Spirit of Truth, when invited to live within our hearts has the power to communicate to us and make us able to know we have remembered correctly. Without having to have anyone else's approval or input. One of my favorite things about following God – He's the only person I ever have to please! If you haven't asked Jesus to live in your heart and be your Savior, Friend, King and Healer, it's super easy, all you have to do is ask. He sees you and thinks you're lovely, He can hear you just believe. It really is that simple.

We need not get obsessed by the recovery of a whole memory. There is much I don't remember and I'm content. Glad, actually! I've known and recovered enough to deal with what needs dealing. There is such a thing as tormenting memories. In this instance, be advised, our Heavenly Father does not torment. The memories He helps you recover may be painful but you will know and feel peace along with them.

5

He will be with you and it will feel like the cleansing of an open wound. Pain with purpose.

Most of us have experienced scrapes that need cleansing. If using hydrogen-peroxide, there's that first jolt of cold and fizzy bubbling discomfort. But it immediately begins to mellow into feeling good. This is what memory recovery with Christ will be like. There will likely be much emotional turmoil surrounding these memories, but God is able to give peace and joy in the midst. If the memories seem to be otherwise, like flashbacks at inappropriate times or with a force that lacks peace, it is a time to plead the blood of Christ over your mind and heart. To hide yourself in Jesus and reject any torment. Maybe move away from the exercise of retrieval for a time to give yourself a chance to do as Psalm 91 advises and get under the shadow of His wings. Our God is a God of peace and love. Be aware.

Psalm 91:4

> *He will cover you with His pinions, and under His wings you may seek refuge; His faithfulness is a shield and bulwark.*

Completely accurate recall of an event is impossible. That's why police investigators want as many witnesses as possible. Each person is observing from a unique spot with a unique filter. Let us not get hung up on 'perfecting' the memory. Holes are likely to be present and some misconception is inevitable. But it's your own memory, for your own healing purposes before God, it should be colored uniquely by you. The only time I recommend being concerned about specific facts is if one must testify in a court of law or if one has made the choice to openly accuse the perpetrator. Otherwise, give yourself permission to believe yourself. Remember, the Holy Spirit, who is also called the Spirit of Truth will be with you. Trust Him.

Okay, I believe the Bible. I believe this can be done. What now?

That's a great question.

The thing that worked best for me was journaling. I felt safe allowing myself to write down whatever humiliating scene flashed in my mind. Along with every disgusting fantasy or self-destructive thought.

It's a place to begin.

Once I had these things down on paper, the substance of memories, and the feelings the memories inspired, seemed smaller. Manageable.

That's good news!

At first, the last thing I wanted to do was write this crap down. Don't let the fear and disgust stop you. Rest in the knowledge that it's only going to become easier and easier.

And believe it!

CHAPTER TWO

Dunamis

M *ay He remember all your sacrifices and accept your
burnt offerings.*
Psalm 20:3

Suggested Oils:

Wild Orange - The oil of abundance

> "It inspires limitless solutions for problems and issues.
> One never needs to live in fear. Wild Orange invites in-
> dividuals to completely let go as a child does and to live
> from their True Self."

Respiratory Blend - The oil of breath

> "They distrust whether it's safe to open and take in life.
> Respiratory blend encourages individuals to release grief
> and sadness and to receive genuine love and healing.
> Respiratory blend also supports one relationship with
> spirit and deepens one's connection to life."

2 Timothy 1:7

> *For God has not given us a spirit of timidity, but of power and love and discipline.*

1 John 4:8

> *There is no fear in love; but perfect love casts out fear, because fear involves punishment and the one who fears is not perfected in love.*

When I began this chapter, the title was 'Fear'. When I went in for the rewrite that title put me off. Looking at the word was building a road-block in my mind and impeding my progress. I want to talk about the fear that is coming, or, most likely, already present. But that's not an accurate description of what this chapter is about. It's actually about overcoming fear and showing it who The Boss is. Jesus! Therefore, the true title of this chapter is meant to be 'Power' because that's exactly what The Spirit of Jesus will give us.

2 Timothy 1:7

> *For God has not given us a spirit of timidity, but of power, and love and discipline.*

Directly from my Bible's Greek word dictionary. Page 2145 1411. dunamis, doo'-nam'is;[2]

Force (literal or figurative); specifically miraculous power (usually by implication, a miracle itself):- ability, abundance, meaning, might (-ily, -y, -y deed), (worker of) miracle (-s), power, strength, violence, might (wonderful) work.

---

[2] Hebrew – Greek Key Word Study Bible NASB 1977 Edition

(B) Generally; a spirit of strength, meaning manly vigor in opposition to a spirit of cowardice.

Let's contrast that with the word timidity. Again, copied directly from my Bible.

Deilia, di-lee'-ah

Timidity, fear. Noun from deilos' fearful. Timid. Cowardice. Timidity. Reticence, fearfulness.

Syn. Deilia is always in a bad sense as contrasted with phobos (5401) fear

Last but not least the word for spirit.

Page 2255

4151 pneuma

B. The rational spirit, mind, body. (2) as referring to the disposition, feeling, temper. Of mind; eg the spirit of gentleness.

The fear, if not already present, is gonna come knockin' and it's no sweetheart. It will pound on the rooftop and rush at you like a suffocating blitz. It's gonna make a lot of noise. But the truth is, fear has no power. Fear gets its power from the individual. It's stalking. It's parasitic. It strikes with the force of your own feelings.

"Forewarned is forearmed."

Fear cannot beat you. Fear cannot stop you. All it can do is inspire emotion. Those emotions may be powerful, but with a little observation, know how, and faith, you can ditch fear for good. I did.

Fear makes me angry because it's a bully. For some of us, it dictates our lives. Sisters, this should not be! Fear will try to control a person and some people allow it. It disturbs me extremely.

So I'm here to repeat what Jesus has said, "Don't be afraid".

John 14:27

> *Peace I leave with you; My peace I give to you; not as the world gives, do I give to you. Let not your heart be troubled, nor let it be fearful.*

Choose His Peace.

Jesus has given us His own peace by His own proclamation. He said flat out, you don't gotta be afraid. Does that seem too easy? After all, there is real and present danger, not to mention evil in this world. God has provided a way for us to deal with legitimate fear worthy situation. He didn't say there's nothing to be afraid of, He said not to allow our hearts to be afraid. We have been given a choice. He also provides power to fulfill our choice. Add discipline to your faith and it becomes a simple exercise in repetition.

Fear is a lie.

Fear is a complete bully. Not cool!

Fear has no place in your life. None.

I'm talking about that fear that pushes you into cowardice. Like when you know you should standup for a person being bullied but you stay hidden in the crowd.

I'm talking about that fear that intimidates you into shirking a duty. Like maybe the duty towards giving yourself a voice in a world that wants to silence the victorious individual.

What about fear that binds you? Like feeling threatened that if you do the right you know you should something bad will happen to you?

I'm talking about that fear that petrifies you into immobility. Like a stagnant life.

It is any fear that infringes on your ability to go boldly forth and be your real true self and by doing that displaying the splendor and handiwork of God. For you, my friend, are His masterpiece.

We have no patience or time for that fear. As soon as it's detected, it needs to be kicked to the curb. And yes, kicked with a violent prejudice. We can do that! I say 'as soon as it's detected' because like the coward it is, it will try to hide so it may keep operating in your life.

We have been given the power to ditch fear forever because God's Word is not simply repetitious, positive thinking. God's Word is living and active and will not return void. God's Word will accomplish what it sets out to do. Every. Single. Time.

Hebrews 4:12

For the Word of God is living and active.

Isaiah 55:11

So is my Word that goes out from my mouth: it will not return to me empty, but will accomplish what I desire and achieve the purpose for which I sent it.

Time may be a factor. It could take time to learn how to skillfully and faithfully wield The Sword of The Spirit and apply it rightly to our lives.

Ephesians 6:17

Take the sword of The Spirit, which is the Word of God.

Charles Spurgeon, who is sometimes regarded as the 19th centuries finest preacher and known as the 'Prince of Preachers' said April 19, 1891:

To be a Christian is to be a warrior. The good soldier of Jesus Christ must not expect to find ease in this world. We have no order from our Captain to patch up a truce, and get as good terms as we can. The one note that rings out from the text is this: TAKE THE SWORD! TAKE THE SWORD!

To take up The Sword of The Spirit and defeat fear will begin with one learning to rightly handle the instrument, God's Word. Making oneself obedient to its Truth.

Psalm 119:11

I have hidden Thy Word in my heart that I might not sin against you.

Psalm 119:105

Thy Word is a lamp unto my feet and a Light unto my path.

Let God's Word renew your mind and transform you. We take a scripture like 1 John 4:18:

There is no fear in love, but perfect love casts out fear. For fear has to do with punishment, and whoever fears has not been perfected in love.

Meditate on His words.

Through reading this scripture, we realize The Truth—that God does not have fear or torment or punishment in His plan for us; therefore, if it is present, it is not of God and we have every right—an obligation even—to use God's Word to force fear out of our lives. It will not go willingly. Again, and this bears repeating, God's Word is not simply positive affirmations. It's Power!

John 8:32

Then you will know the truth and the truth will set you free.

`Psalm 31:4, 5, 21, 24

Thou wilt pull me out of the net which they have secretly laid for me: For Thou art my strength. Into Thy hand I commend my spirit; Thou hast ransomed me, O Lord, God of Truth.

Blessed be The Lord, for He has made marvelous His loving kindness to me in a besieged city.

Be strong and let your heart take courage, all you who hope in The Lord.

You've got to make a choice, will you let your heart take courage?

Do you know what you're afraid of?

Sometimes when I have aired my fears aloud, that alone revealed their inherent ridiculousness and they dissipated simply from that exercise. Other times I've had to hold on strenuously to a piece of God's Word, repeat it out loud just to believe it, then keep it in front of me until it saturated the soil of my heart as it acted dually as a poison to suffocate the weeds of lies, thick and menacing, and at the same time raising up banners of victorious Truth like marigolds. Vibrant, cheerful, sturdy. But I had to choose to take hold and hang on!

List your fears. Search God's Word for that scripture passage that illuminates, by the power of the Holy Spirit, and grasp that verse until its Truth and power is your default setting. And the lie is utterly extinct.

Start with your concordance and look up verses on fear. See where that leads.

There are Biblical Promises handbooks that make finding applicable scriptures easier. As well as spiritual warfare books that will help fill your arsenal. It almost doesn't matter what scripture verse you use. God's Word dispels darkness. Your enemy of fear cannot stand in The Light of God's Word. Use it!

2 Timothy 3: 16,17

> *All scripture is God-breathed and is useful for teaching, rebuking, correcting, and training in righteousness. So that the servant of God may be thoroughly equipped for every good work.*

All scripture is breathed from God's own mouth. How much actual power it contains may possibly depend on how much you can believe. Believe big, ladies! He is The Almighty! All Mighty. He is able. He is!

He wants to move on your behalf. He is mindful of you, sweet girl. For a girl, whose body and heart has been violated by the violent dominance lust visits on her, opening oneself and trusting enough to allow God's power to enter in and begin to remove the hurt, takes a faith bigger than average. Especially because as John 15 informs us, *He is The Vinedresser and He cuts off every branch that bears no fruit.* Further, He prunes every branch that does bear fruit to be even more fruitful. As a child of sexual abuse, I had many branches bearing no fruit, or worse, rotten fruit. In the beginning, it just felt like a lot of cutting. And that hurts, ya'll. But I believed, and still believe, He has my ultimate best in His mind. There was nowhere else to turn. I don't believe any other has my ultimate best in mind, they just cannot. They are people. And I'm people. God alone knows how to love the individual perfectly. Therefore, I was willing to endure. That hope, like Jesus had, will sustain you!

Hebrews 12:2

Looking unto Jesus, the Author and Finisher of our faith, who for the joy that was set before Him endured the cross, despising the shame, and is set down at the right hand of God.

There's a cross to carry. But it will not be more than you can bear. Check out 1 Corinthians 10:13. This verse is about temptation, and how when the cutting starts you may be tempted towards unbelief. Hold fast the Word of hope, and remember the joy of your goal which is having the consistency and wholeness to live the life of which you've been dreaming! He will uphold you with His Righteous Right Hand!

A word about shame.

Jesus despised the shame of public humiliation and rejection.

Despise: to regard with contempt, distaste, disgust, or disdain: scorn; loathe.

Scorn: open or unqualified contempt; disdain.

Contempt: the feeling with which a person regards anything considered mean, vile, or worthless; disdain; scorn.

Disdain: to look upon or treat with contempt; despise; scorn.

Girls, I'm convinced shame is a worthless feeling. If we allow it to influence us it will make us hide. Hiding is not the answer.

Shame is not a tool of our Heavenly Father.

Jeremiah 31:3

> *The Lord appeared to us in the past, saying: 'I have loved you with an everlasting love; I have drawn you with unfailing kindness.'*

Shame is part and parcel to sin, sin done to us and sin we commit. But we do not need to cling to it. Do not believe the shame. It will convince you quickly you're worthless and how could God (or anyone) love you. It is a lie! Our enemy is the father of lies. Let us never agree with him in Jesus' name!

John 8:44

> *…he was a murderer from the beginning, not holding to the Truth, for there is no truth in him. When he lies, he speaks his native language, for he is a liar and the father of lies.*

1 Peter 5:8

> *Be alert and sober minded. Your enemy the devil prowls around like a roaring lion looking for someone to devour.*

Our enemy would petrify us with his roars. For it is the only way he may catch us. If he can scare us or make us feel shame enough to hide from The Light of Jesus then we put ourselves in a position of being sitting ducks. Let's not use our God given power to run into the enemies trap.

Instead:

Hebrews 10:23

Let us hold fast the profession of our faith without wavering; for He is Faithful that promised.

1 Thessalonians 5:24

The One who calls you is Faithful, and He will do it.

John 14:4

You may ask me for anything in my Name, and I will do it.

James 1:6,7

But when you ask, you must believe and not doubt, because the one who doubts is like a wave of the sea, blown and tossed by the wind. That person should not expect to receive anything from The Lord.

I have this picture in my mind, like a cartoon of a small child on her knees before a huge lion. This lion roars right in her face and we can see the force by the blowing of her hair and quivering of her flesh. But she hunkers down. Once the roar has ended, once it's gone, the lion follows. He crumbles into dust and is blown away by the true might of the presence of the Holy Spirit.

The roar of shame will endeavor to push you into hiding. Be wise and alert. Once detected get your Sword, God's

Word, and send that malarkey back to hell where it belongs. It does not belong on you. God Himself has said loving kindness belongs on you. Those are His tools of choice. In them you will obtain healing and rest.

CHAPTER THREE

Rejection

*M*ay He give you the desire of your heart and make all
your plans succeed.
Psalm 20:4

Suggested Oils:

Roman Chamomile - The oil of spiritual purpose

"Roman Chamomile assists a person in shedding the
meaningless activities that consume their lives, so they
can focus on more fulfilling work, even the work of their
own souls. This oil assists in feeling connected to and
supported by divine helpers and guides, and calms insecurities about following one's spiritual path."

Bergamot -The oil of self-acceptance

"Bergamot teaches individuals to let go of self-judge-
ment by learning to love themselves unconditionally."

Birch - The oil of support

"This oil offers courage to move forward alone."

Check out 1 Peter 2:4, 5

Rejection. I've gone round and round with this one. It always seems to take the heart right out of me. Then I lose the battle. It hurts to be rejected. To feel small. To be made to feel worthless by others. It's mean and it's cruel and the message that we are not wanted comes through loud and clear. This is the one that gets me. Fear, no problem. I'll knock that out every time. Easy. But people disliking me? I am already so fragile, already believing myself all kinds of ugly, and so desperately dependent on the kindness of those around me to help me believe I'm okay and I want to live. Then they confirm all my worst thoughts about myself by not wanting me around. It's like nothing to them. But to me, it's like the gavel dropping, the judgement is decided. It's true. I am worthless. Unlovable. Unaccepted. Undesirable. All the yucky stuff.

But I'm not built to run or quit. Besides, my brain believes God's Word even though my heart is a flood of despondent emotions. I have a skill to step outside my feelings and observe what's happening to me. It's been a very useful tool. Probably what's kept me from utter ruin. Well, God's love has accomplished that because apart from it there is no hope.

With my observation skill I can see the feelings brought on by rejection are just that, feelings in response to others' opinions. However, from those feelings, I've constructed beliefs about what's really true regarding my worth and the importance of having a proper family. Feelings, created in response to a lie, is like adding a thick fog over a hedge maze. Using our feelings, feelings that have been born of abuse, to decide what's really true… Using feelings that resulted from abuse to decide what's true? 'Truth' manufactured by feelings in response to abuse will always warp the worldview. And is no truth at all.

My rejection outline:

1. Somebody hurt me

2. Somebody rejected me

3. Hurt feelings flooded

4. Beliefs developed

5. Behaviors followed beliefs

What does your rejection look like? Can you identify it? What about beliefs that stem from it? Behaviors?

For me, I was rejected by family. Now when I see what I perceive as 'a good family', it makes me believe I've lost something so valuable it cannot be replaced. Which is true, my blood family is lost to me. Real relationships and years that could have been filled with joy and love are gone. Bitterness grows in my heart. My negative feelings open the door for beliefs to be established, which prepare the way for bitterness to grow, which creates more bad feelings that deepen and confirm the beliefs and so on.

I'm really up the creek without a paddle. What hope is there? What resolution is there that may satisfy a broken heart? There is a way. It's narrow but doable!

U-turn! I'm super stoked because once I took the whole 'rejection' issue as something real, once the fruit of this hidden misconception began to grow up and interrupt my life, finally, I then sought The Lord to show me how to deal with this loss. To be clear, the loss is real. The disintegration of the family is a serious blow both to the individual and society in general, but also to the witness and image of God's glory, power and love. I say again, the loss is real. The sorrow from such loss is completely warranted and perfectly legitimate. To not have bad feelings from such loss would be disturbing. Embrace, accept and allow yourself the luxury of being true.

What's the stoked part? This is where it gets exciting. In the reality of heaven, there is no such thing as loss. This world is set up to function one way, and our bodies being dust of the earth, connect us intimately to this world system. But our spirits belonging to God, redeemed by God, gives us ability and access to rise above the temporal to know, believe, and focus our energies on the things above.

I want to accept my circumstances and feelings for what they are. More importantly, I want to know God's Word and make this the habitation of my thoughts, treasures and hopes.

So, what does God's Word say to me [us] about rejection?

First, I gotta hit up Psalm 71 and give snaps to one of my spiritual mothers, Mrs. Nick. I got mad love for ya for sending me to Psalm 71 when I asked her what scriptures came to her mind regarding the issue of rejection.

When we read the Word of God, amazing things can happen. The Holy Spirit will illuminate for us what we are reading so our minds are able to comprehend The Word; but even more magical is he makes it applicable in so unique a way, so very intimate. It's thrilling and like receiving the most wholesome meal on the stormiest and hungriest day.

Wonderful revelations were given to me from reading Psalm 71.

Recently, in my home, for my two-year-old son, I got guinea pigs, a rabbit, four chickens and a dog. The appropriate habitat has become a topic of interest and study. The wrong habitat is deadly. To my shame, I almost froze our guinea pigs to death by not moving them back into the house for winter sooner. Like a slipshod meteorologist, which is my training in the USAF, I was reading Celsius and thinking Fahrenheit. They can't survive at temperatures below 60 degrees Fahrenheit. So, at 4 am one September morning, I was frantically figuring a space for them indoors when it was forty-two degrees Fahrenheit outside. But they lived and are fat and happy (as all piggies should be). When I read Psalm 71:3 "Be Thou to me a Rock of Habitation" I immediately thought:

> *God is my Habitat.*

It makes so much sense! He is my whole home, my whole world. It is deadly to dwell, or even step outside that habitat. I'm more like a guinea pig than I may want to admit. It does give me comfort though. It was like heaving a sigh of relief to imagine myself living, playing, traveling, sleeping, and working in the habitat God Himself, has designed specifically for me. Just for me.

Next verse 6 jumped out at me.

> *By Thee I have been sustained from birth;*
> *Thou art He who took me from my mothers womb;*
> *My praise is continually of Thee.*

The idea: it is God, not parents, Who sustains me. That idea came to me in bright flashing lights causing this darkness covering my mind to become glittery dust, and be gone.

This is the core thought of my rejection issues:

My parents don't love me. Nobody loves me. I can never replace my parents. I will never have that love. I will always have a hole. Dark. Cold. Lonely. And I must be ugly to have been forsaken.

This line of thought has been operating in my heart and life for at least thirty-three years. Like guerrilla warfare, it's been operating and hiding in the shadows of my heart. Its effectiveness relies on secrecy. I have no idea what the sum of damage this particular lie has grown in my life. Every bit of self-destruction I pursued has some smack of this stench on it.

Yet in the moment God's Word was given to me, empowered by the Holy Spirit and my meager efforts to believe, the lie dissolved. The secrecy and darkness is paramount to its survival. In The Light of God's Word, it shriveled up and was gone. It. Could. Not. Stand. In. His. Light. Simply put, God has sustained me from the beginning. Always and all ways. I do not require the love or participation of those who've rejected me. The original reality, the Truth behind the masquerade, is God wants me. Made me. Loves me. He goes to great lengths to demonstrate this to me. And He has never left me. He is my Habitat. That's all I need. Sometimes it really feels like a sweet gift to not have parents. Sometimes they can be a hinderance to becoming who we are meant to be in Christ. They could possibly block our view and need of our Heavenly Father. So I focus on His Truth. I walk in it. I'm thankful. It works.

Next verse: Psalm 71:14

> *But as for me, I will hope Continually,*
> *And will praise Thee yet more And more.*

I will! I will hope continually!

Continually: adverb 1. very often; at regular or frequent intervals; habitually.

That hope pulls me through many a dark place. both in my heart and in the world.

Praise. God inhabits His people when they praise. His Presence will manifest sooner or later in praise. Sometimes it has not been sensually discernible, still, healing occurred. Therefore, He was present. Had the healing been delayed, still He is there. But keep praising. No darkness can endure in His Presence.

Next Verse: Psalm 71:15

> *My mouth shall tell of They Righteousness*
> *And of Thy Salvation all day Long;*
> *For I do not know the sum of Them.*

It's interesting to think of how many aspects of God we miss out on by not talking about them. If I am going to talk about them, I must first be thinking about them. How important, for our thoughts to revolve around Him. His attributes. Beauty. What He has done. Will do. My own thoughts are toxic when I let them run free—ranging from grandiose ideas down to paranoid, make-believe conversations. But He really will keep in perfect peace my mind (my life as a result, relationships, finances, health) when it dwells on Him. Isaiah 26:3 informs us of this Truth. Because we trust in Him, because we certainly can trust Him. Think of Him. Our thoughts make or break us.

Next verse: Psalm 71:17

> *O God, Thou hast taught me*
> *From my youth.*

He wants to guide. Give Him that chance.

Next verse: Psalm 71:24

> *For they are ashamed, for they*
> *Are humiliated who seek*
> *My hurt.*

At first, it's like, yeah God, get 'em! Get 'em good! Enjoy your just desserts. But darn it, I Corinthians 13 comes to mind and I'm reminded that love does not delight in evil but rejoices with the truth. It's to my benefit to understand, accept, and practice this word from God. It isn't right to be glad for another's harm.

However, we may hope for and rejoice over justice. Once we really receive healing from God. Once the depth of my own depravity and offenses against God were realized, it becomes important that God loves us all. That there is hope even for those who have mortally wounded us. He forgives and He empowers us through His Spirit to also forgive and be free. Still, justice remains.

Let's take a moment to dwell on forgiveness.

Romans 5:8

> *But God demonstrates His own love for us in this: while we were still sinners, Christ died for us.*

I have only one son. To give him up to a bunch of ungrateful, evil people who will assuredly beat, humiliate, and kill him: no. it's completely outside of the realm of possibility. I would not sacrifice my son. Thank you, God, you have already done the really hard parts for us. He does for us the parts we cannot do for ourselves.

Romans 3:23

> *For all have sinned and fall short of the glory of God.*

Isaiah 64:6

> *All of us have become like one who is unclean, and all our righteous acts are like filthy rags; we all shrivel up like a leaf, and like the wind our sins sweep us away.*

God's Word is perfect. The truth is, I ain't got no room to talk about condemning another. Just as soon as I do all my filthy rags rise up and bear witness exclaiming:

"Who are you?"

We all sin. All sin is exactly the same. Except for sexual sin and blasphemy (1 Corinthians 6:18/Matthew 12:31, 32 respectively). God levels the playing field. It is only us who categorize sin and tries to act like our excrement doesn't offend the olfactory sense. Everyone. Every single individual has no platform to stand on if one wants to accuse and condemn another. Don't worry about what happens to the other guy. We are all working out our own salvation. I cannot hurt you without hurting myself. Justice will prevail. All those traitors to humanity are earning their just rewards, even if we cannot see it. God does not let anything slip. Not even a sparrow falls to the ground but that He is mindful of it. There is no good old boys club with Him. He will not show favoritism. But that's His biz. I gotta leave it to Him. That's trust. That's faith.

Traitors to humanity. Indeed, betraying even their own identity. An act of exerting one's power over another in order to dominate, violate, and take what hasn't been given is a choice in the affirmative to become a cannibalistic beast, a thing that preys upon it's own kind and by that practice becomes less and less human. It is death. It is destruction. It is hell on earth. There isn't language foul enough to classify these acts. But if we are true, we can see that most of us, to some degree, are seeking to exert dominance over another individual on the daily. We're all capable of becoming beastly. We need our wholeness to create heaven on earth where redemption exists. Even for that vile cannibal thief if he would be made new.

Think of this:

Matthew 6:15

> *But if you do not forgive others their sins, your Father will not forgive your sins.*

Zounds! Cause for pause. Don't even worry about this. I hear the cries;

> *I can never forgive! Neither will I!*

We all, before we can forgive others need work in our own hearts. Mortal wounds are what we receive when we have been violated sexually. Imagine seeing every girl who's been raped, or worse, walking around town with her belly sliced open and she's got her own entrails in one hand. It looks like bloody murder. Nobody is going to ask that girl to run a marathon. Nobody is going to ask her to go and fetch them a glass of water. Somebody who is healthy will take that girl to the hospital. To me, that's what's happening all over. We've taken mortal wounds, but they are on the inside. So, what? They don't count? Think of the girl holding her entrails, make-up on and trying to smile, going through life trying to make everyone else comfortable by denying her wound and being okay. God knows right where I am. He isn't gonna ask me to do something He won't give me power to accomplish. Just accept His forgiveness. Be made new. Later on, we can ask God for the will to forgive, even if we never feel like it.

Back to rejection. P.S. I love you so much. I can't help it. "let the kickdrum kick one time, breathe out let your mind unwind, eyes on the ceiling, looking for the feeling, wide open let your own eyes shine." #Switchfoot4ever

Psalm 71

The verses I highlighted; the Holy Spirit illuminated to me as I read this Psalm. It was liberating and joyful and healing.

1 Corinthians 2:14

John 1:9/John 14:26

The Holy Spirit will teach us. He speaks to me through The Word.

While I was reading this Psalm, these scriptures were jumping out at me and rearranging my understanding. There were other thoughts above these, like a two tiered cake. Pictures and ideas were playing scenes and presenting ideas that were also exciting. The main thrust of these ideas was: Jesus was rejected too.

While I was being liberated from the bondage of emotional turmoil regarding rejection through Psalm 71. God was also showing me another aspect of The Truth. Another understanding. He showed me an appropriate point of meditation for the individual grappling with rejection. I believe my feelings to be valid and true. However, I do well to remember feelings aren't facts. Realizing feelings aren't facts opens a whole new kettle of fish. Without invalidating my feelings, I'm willing to concede that my interpretation as a child is not completely accurate of certain behaviors of others. Only God really knows the truth of everyone's hearts. Every individual is operating from a platform of their own hurts, sins, convictions, desires, etc. My feelings are legitimate and deserve to be treated with respect. However, it's also possible those feelings were formed from false information. I'm so thankful for God's Word! He effectively took care of my personal feelings, then led my by the hand into further understanding. My experience is colored through with missing information, warped perceptions, and my own sin. God's Word is not. Therefore, it's a perfect place to find rest. A break from myself. His Word offers complete Truth we can bank on. What a relief to turn my focus away from myself.

The Holy Spirit called to mind Mark 3:32-35

And a multitude was sitting around Him, and they said to Him 'Behold your mother and your brothers are outside looking for you.' And answering them, He said, 'Who are my mother and my brothers! For whoever does the will of God, he is my brother and sister and mother.'

Guess what? I've been born again into God's family. I'm chosen by Him and a co-heir with Christ (Ephesians 1:3, 4/Romans 8:17) I don't even have to care anymore if I don't want to about the worldly 'loss'. None of it even has anything to do with me. People who've rejected me or hurt me weren't treating me according to an educated, informed, critical analysis of my actual worth. That's only possible for God to do and He's already declared we are worth more than we can imagine. No. Those people were responding to their own hurts, angers, perversions and whatever issues hidden in the dark recesses of their hearts. I was just nearby. So, let it go. I don't want to give those circumstances and resulting feelings any long-term care and energy. Yes, I gotta face 'em and deal and forgive and all the steps. But the magnitude can diminish. I can just focus directly, and manage all my feelings, beliefs, and energies within the habitat of God's Presence. Certain things don't have to matter. That just makes me so happy.

The Spirit called to mind two other verses regarding rejection:

Here's the first verse:

Luke 10:16

The one who listens to you listens to Me, and the one who rejects you rejects Me; and he who rejects Me rejects The One who sent me.

Jesus speaking here says, 'Check it, we're in on this together now. You're rejected, cast out, discarded by that one? Me too. Then we go together. Further, they've chosen to reject God, The Father.'

This type of loyalty is revolutionary. Jesus never leaves us or forsakes us. He is the only one who may make that claim. He alone has the power to remain by our side. No matter how much I may desire in my heart to stick by a person, forces outside my control (and that describes basically every force) can at any moment push me out of this world. But nothing and no one has the power to force Jesus to do anything. He is always with me by His own proclamation and desire.

Check out Deuteronomy 31:6.

What do we do with those situations when people have rejected us? Breathe. Breathe. Breathe.

Zephaniah 3:17

Look at The Holy One. He will quiet my heart with His love.

We let it go. We let them go. We forgive. We accept the frailty of others as we accept our own. Remembering the God who sees my sin forgives me, loves me, and also loves those who've hurt us. He knows all my ugliest uglies and still loves me. When I first realized this, it was a bit offensive. He asks me to be like Him. But not on my own hook. He comes through for me. Healing me. Helping me. Showing me His way. The way of true and just Love. He enables me. Suddenly my hurt, abandonment, or rejection isn't a focus.

There's room now to live differently. I would have Him make me to love like Him.

2nd Verse.

Matthew 21:42

> *Jesus said to them, 'Did you never read in the scriptures? The*
> *stone which the builders rejected This became the Chief Corner-*
> *stone; The came about from The Lord, and it is marvelous in our*
> *eyes.'*

Jesus is that stone. Jesus was, is, and will be, rejected by men.
The very people He left glory to come be with, rejected
Him. They didn't love Him. They hated Him. Despised His
Authority. Power. And especially His Love. This love of His
that included whores, tax collectors, the dregs of society. It
seems to me, apart from God, we are all whores. We're all
whoring for something. We just don't appreciate someone
bringing that to light, at all. Exposure! Nothing' Brighter
than Jesus Christ, our Lord. We got to shut that Light down
hard. 'Do not come in here exposing me, Jesus!'

Fear. Again. We don't gotta be afraid of the Light. First of
all, He already knows all about you. Last of all, He's declared
His love for you, with full knowledge of you. His opinion is
the only one that matters.

Jesus was rejected. So how did He handle that? He was not
moved. He did no dancing for people. He stood in that spot
of rejection and trusted God, His Father. Our Father. Keeping His eyes ever on the goal. How did our Father respond
to that? He made Jesus Chief. Whole building falls down if
not for Him.

I have this idea that if I can be like Jesus in this area, keep
my eyes on my Father in heaven, trust him…

By trust I mean believe that this rejection will not define my
life. Believe that His love and acceptance is enough to heal
my desperate places of oozing need. Believe that He will

33

sustain me and walk me through this into a better place. No matter how dark it seems to get I still believe.

If I can do that. If I can handle rejection like Jesus did, I mean, if I rely on Jesus to give me the power and grace to handle rejection like He did, I'm comin' out as a chief. Somehow, some way. Not The Chief of what Jesus is Chief of, only He can do that. But a Little Chief of something. I want that! I believe He is willing and able to do this with me, for me, through me. Steady on, girl!

CHAPTER FOUR

Pleasure

*M*ay we shout for joy over your victory and lift up our banners in the Name of our God. May the Lord grant all your requests. Psalm 20:5

Suggested Oils:

Cinnamon - The oil of sexual harmony

"Cinnamon invites individuals to be honest and vulnerable, thereby allowing true intimacy to emerge."

Rose - The oil of divine love

"It supports individuals in reaching heavenward and connecting with divine love. If one can simply let go and choose to receive divine love, they are wrapped in warmth, charity, and compassion."

I believe God intended it to be the undercurrent of our entire lives. Because of it, He created us. Soon, by His own hand and breath He will carry us to a place He has prepared, specifically, for us, that is forever pleasure—always and only.

Hard to believe when we see beached whales. Children being yelled at. Or hearing that another baby elephant has been orphaned. Another family torn apart by drugs. Another husband and wife divorcing. Does the list end?

Why is pleasure apart of this conversation?

Our goal is to feel good!

If we aren't going to feel better after all the labor intensive, soul searching and prayer and discipline of sorting through the affects and deposits of trauma in our lives, then why do it? If my choices and thinking aren't going to change to produce an over-all improvement of my understanding, relationships, and life; then I'm not doing it.

Does God even care if I feel good?

What precisely do I like?

What makes me feel good?

First, I must stop and pray. This topic is too wonderful for me. Perhaps, that's why we don't hear too much about pleasure, it seems, in the church generally. The topic is befuddling by it's sheer size. And feeling too good sounds dangerous and anti-holy.

Holy Spirit, Spirit of Truth, Spirit of Jesus, Thank You. Thank You for Your attention and Presence. Attend all who read this and enlighten them and me now with a clear understanding and vision of how your plan and work is all pleasurable. Thank You, Spirit. Amen.

Psalm 16:11

Thou wilt make known to me the path of life; In Thy Presence is fulness of joy; In Thy right hand are pleasures forevermore.

When I first became acquainted with Psalm 16:11 it blew me away. My heart instantly jumped up and said YES! to 'pleasures forevermore'. Another translation says 'eternal pleasures'. I really like to use the 'eternal pleasures' measuring stick when I'm going in for something that's gonna feel good.

For me, historically, I like to numb down. Party down. One drink one hit off the ganja pipe—that's never interested me. I want to get fully loaded. Go ballistic. Get louder. Go faster. And putting a stop to alcohol and weed was not a decision I wanted to make in the affirmative. I asked God to change my heart.

I prayed:

Lord, You know I don't want to stop smoking weed. You gotta change my heart and mind Man. I'm not gonna be able to do it.

My self was emotionally and physically attached to getting high. But my intellectual mind knew it wasn't really delivering what it promised.

HIGH IS A LIE!

What's left for a girl to do? Continue on til I've convinced myself the lie is true? Not this kid. I have a will. Maybe it's not strong enough to stop a growing dependence on mind altering substance. But it's strong enough to simply ask The Lord for help. Just between me and Him. No intervention. No weirdness. Just a humble request and a quiet belief He loves me enough to respond. He did. He changed my heart. And now, sometimes a nostalgia of romanticized memories of how good it feels to get high approaches me and I begin to consider picking up a pipe. I have a great pipe. It's long, like a wizard might possess. But. I start thinking about what getting high is actually gonna do. Maybe a temporary, fleeting, good feeling. But, eventually, it's not gonna feel good. There's lung pollution to consider. Coming down. How will it affect those around me? An eternal pleasure feels good before, during and after the action on into eternity.

Have any of us been involved in illicit affairs? Before beginning one ask: will this feel good before, during and after, on into eternity? A bad love making session with my husband could be all kinds of things—disappointing, irritating, an unwanted bother, a duty—but it still meets the before, during and on into eternity criteria. An amazing, mind blowing, indescribably sexy and sensuous sex session with a man not my husband does not meet the criteria. Nor can it. Ever.

Let's feel good, girls! Let's begin to ask ourselves: Does this cookie feel good now? Will it feel good later? If the answer is no at any point on the timeline let's ask God to help us take our hands off it and move them to eternal pleasures. Something that feels good all the way through.

Now these are just examples. Not all weed use is wrong. There is no loophole for sex outside of marriage. That's always going to be wrong. Some cookie eating in life is not only okay but probably essential. You, standing before God, will know what, for you, is an eternal pleasure. Get before Him. Let Him surprise you with true pleasure. He will sustain you with pleasure to pleasure. You won't even be able to imagine how that's possible until one day, you look around, and you're surrounded by eternal pleasures. There will still be work to be done, still the upsets and complications and more work, but suddenly, cleaning up the full cup of coffee my two year old son spilled at 0537 hours by running through the house, hollering because he's too full of joy and life to realize it's time for quiet coffee and waking up, and I'm so annoyed as I mop up my coffee. And the noise. At that moment my heart thanks god for the privilege of having husband, home and child. Still takes me thirty minutes to get my head clear. I still need a break from my work. But my heart is thankful and glad. It's pretty cool my friend. Those eternal pleasure suit me. What will yours look like? You should write to me and tell me. And especially once they all manifest.

Remember too in His Presence is fulness of joy. Might still be sobbing and heart broken, but that's not the foundation, atmosphere nor ultimate outcome. He transports us from glory to glory. In His presence is fulness of joy. In His Presence is fulness of joy. In His Presence is fulness of joy.

For pleasure, use your measuring stick. Is this an eternal pleasure?

I pray:

> Lord, Father God, help me.

What makes me feel good?

What excites me?

What stirs and thrills my heart?

Zephaniah 3: 12-20

> *But I will leave among you*
> *A humble and lowly people,*
> *And they will take refuge in*
> *The Name of The Lord*
>
> *The remnant of Israel will*
> *Do no wrong*
> *And tell no lies*
> *Nor will a deceitful tongue*
> *Be found in their mouths;*

For they shall feed and lie
Down
With no one to make them
Tremble.

Shout for joy, O daughter of
Zion!
Shout in triumph, O Israel!
Rejoice and exult with all your
Heart.
O daughter of Jerusalem!

Take a moment to visualize how you'd live if you were
fearless.

The Lord has taken away
His judgement against you,
He has cleared away your
Enemies.

The King of Israel, The Lord,
Is in your midst;
You will fear disaster no
More.

In that day it will be said to
Jerusalem:
Do not be afraid, O Zion;
Do not let your hands fall
Limp,
The Lord you God is
In your midst,
A Victorious Warrior.
He will exult over you with joy,
He will be quiet in His love,
He will rejoice over you with
Shouts of joy.

I will gather those who
Grieve about the appointed
Feasts

They came from you O Zion;
The reproach of exile is a
Burden on them.
Behold, I am going to deal
At that time
With all your oppressors.
I will save the lame
And gather the outcast,
And I will turn their
Shame into praise and
Renown
In all the earth.
He is present. Worship Him!

'At that time I will bring you in,
Even at the time hen I gather
You together;
Indeed, I will give you
Renown and praise
Among all the peoples of the
Earth.
When I restore your
Fortunes, before your
Eyes, '
Says The Lord.

Some Bible scholars and theologians will say these verses are not for us. They are spoken to a certain people for a certain time. I humbly beg to differ. God does what he wants. If His Holy Spirit chooses to illuminate particular verses to me personally through His Own Word, then I'm not trying to get technical with The Almighty and remind

Him to please be reasonable and more believable and basically try to cut Him down to my size. Heck. To. The. No. I'm takin it!

This study is personal. Reading God's Word is intimate. He wants us to know Him. To be able to understand and accept His love. Knowing too, that while he shouts for joy over us, like we just read, He is also the Vinedresser, and with His love cuts off everything in me that bears no fruit. (John 15) Does that sound painful? It's so easy to believe the painful part and grow bitter towards Him. I want us to believe bigger in His ecstatic joy for us that causes Him to shout about us. Me. You. The individual.

Pleasure: enjoyment or satisfaction derived from what is to one's liking; gratification; delight.

There were many things God spoke to me through Zephaniah 3:12-20. I wonder, what is He speaking to you?

Much of what He spoke is for me personally. Which I may someday share. Specifically, for this work, presently, verse 14 has been my focus.

> *Shout for joy*
> *O daughter of Zion!*
> *Should in triumph*
> *O Israel!*
> *Rejoice and exult*
> *With*
> *All your heart,*
> *O daughter of Jerusalem!*

I really wanted to put myself to the test and measure my ability to have a fully exultant heart. I know God is speaking directly to me asking me to simply be joyful. Make the choice to allow myself to shout for joy. It sounds like I should be anxious to receive this instruction from The Lord.

And how easy to follow through and accomplish, yet, I really wasn't too glad about it. Immediately I could feel my inability to let myself go. Truly. Sincerely. With naked, vulnerable, honesty before God, or, in my family life to get an energetic joy. Energy is required for the joy shout. Supernatural energy! Can't shout without the energy. I could quietly be joyful in my heart. Part of it. Some places in myself I refuse to let joy in. Or the energy.

Check out Nehemiah 8:10.

Why? We all have our reasons. It may be necessary to identify and analyze reasons. It may not be for some. However, we get there, the answer to possessing the supernatural energy for a joy shout is walking with Christ through our days.

I was walking through my garage to get my bunny some timothy hay when Jesus told me the answer to healing those places, I'd refused joy. I'd been asking Him throughout the day. I was looking for a verse and a speedy resolution. I came to know the places I would not allow the joy was my belly and bowels. My whole visceral section, responsible for digesting in the literal and spiritual sense has been refusing the energy and Light of God. Uhm, that's bad. The next chapter will go deeper in the belly business. But right now, to begin, the answer is found in Matthew 17:21.

Matthew 17: 21

But this kind does not go out except by prayer and fasting.

Jesus is speaking to the disciples here explaining why a laying on of their hands and commands could not expel the evil spirit. Okay. So now we know, this is gonna require a participation and discipline from us. A cooperation with Christ. Jesus also said, "When you fast…" (Matthew 6:16) not if you fast. I get 'hangry'. If I don't eat, I get super

43

grouchy! God has always been so kind to me regarding fasting. If I have intended to fast one meal or a certain food item instead of a lengthy, pious nuthin' but water fast, He's come through for me. Your fasting, my fasting, is completely personal. Let the Holy Spirit guide you.

Here's a worthy question.

Do I want to shout for joy? Am I willing for God to lead me through the work to get to that holy energized exultant heart? Yes! I am. Are you? I couldn't perform the actions of obedience to God's Word straight away. Once I agreed with Him (He gives freewill, it's my choice!) I needed to ask Him to help me begin to walk in an exultant heart. Seemingly weird, that started in my guts with fasting. The link? Surrendered heart, I'm practicing. Fulfilling God's Word takes God's own power in our lives. Even something like being joyful, which at first glance seems totally counterintuitive. We cannot be joyful on our own. We need Him if we are ever to live our lives in true joy and be able to break out with a true triumphant victoriously joyful shout!

Ask God today, this very moment agree, and ask Him to show you where you're holding back, where you're hiding. Ask Him to bring His Light and joy to those places. Begin to allow yourself the strength of joy.

Are you still uncertain The Almighty esteems pleasure as a priority in our lives? Look at The Song of Songs. He's included in His Word an entire book about desire. Anticipation. Obsession even. And gratification. Look at His world. He's created an extremely provocative display of sensuous pleasure. Filled with sights, sounds, smells and feels designed to give clean intoxication to the body. Thus, inspiring and enhancing a lifting of the spirit. The smell of the ocean. It's salty spray. The sound of the waves, gulls and what else? Just one example. Look at the flowers. Meditate on their perfection. Softness. Some force in them that insists on blooming in rocky places yet still regal with fragility.

Like us, ladies. Clothed in soft fragility, yet capable of carrying the heaviest loads for great distances with aplomb. Is there anything more pleasurable than the human female form? With her tender strength. Soft curves. Steel devotion. Healing touch. Creative mind. A heart built to love.

Ephesians 1:5

> *Having predestined us unto the adoption of children by Jesus Christ to Himself, according to the good pleasure of His will.*

He does what feels good. Let's be like Him.

CHAPTER FIVE

Belly

*N*ow this I know: The Lord gives victory to His anointed.
He answers him from His heavenly sanctuary with the
victorious power of His right hand. Psalm 20:6

Suggested Oils:

Ginger - The oil of empowerment

> "Ginger empowers individuals in taking complete re-
> sponsibility for their life circumstances. It infuses a war-
> rior-like mentality based on integrity, personal responsi-
> bility, and individual choice."

Fennel - The oil of responsibility

> "Fennel reignites a passion for life. Fennel reestablishes
> a strong connection to the body and the self when there
> has been weakness or separation. Fennel also supports
> an individual in listening to the subtle messages of the
> body."

Belly time. Sa-weet! Everyone loves their belly. But naught.
I recently read Giulia Enders book, *GUT.* What a great

work! She talks about the fact that when we are beginning to be formed in the womb by God (I added the God part) every time He starts us out the same way. Basically, three tubes form first. The tubes that make up the brain, the heart and the belly. C.S. Lewis says, "Put first things first and second things are thrown in. Put second things first and you lose both first and second things."

In forming the physical that reflects the unseen, God puts our hearts, brains and guts first. As Christians we are hip to the renewing of our minds. Let's keep it cerebral people! Some of us are into the heart and how Proverbs 23:7 tells us that as a man thinketh in his heart so he is. We have gleaned the understanding we may also think from our hearts.

What we've been missing, or strategically blinded to is that our guts have been given intelligence by The Most High as well. We aren't talking about gluttony as a sin. A deadly sin. And is for many. We aren't discussing the meaning and implications or dangers of Philippians 3:19 that confirms for some, their stomach is their god. Jesus says 'not if but when you fast. He also, when instructing the disciples taught them some evil spirits will come out only by prayer and fasting. Daniel and the lions. We all know the victory God gave him by shutting up the mouths of the lions. How many of us are as excited about Daniel and his three pals refusing the kings victuals? Was there more to that than physical health? Did that represent a spiritual health as well? Maybe that opened the door for Daniel to be so intimate with God he had no hesitation of going against all society to bow down three times a day in public view. What about the confidence to descend into a lair of lions?

Girls, we can no longer afford to ignore our bellies. Or gloss over that our guts too are a legitimate part of the image He has created to appear, somehow, like Him. Our guts represent some aspect of Him. He created our digestive system specifically. Purposefully. And He called our bodies a good work. (Genesis 1:31) He has said we are made with respect, reverence, and wonder!

Our tummies have just as major a role to play in our recovery and healing as our brains and hearts. For every man. Especially for those who've endured trauma. Our digestive systems are super trainable. We are malleable and moldable. Like clay. Our Heavenly Father is The Master Craftsman and Creator. However, we are made to be like Him. We have been given some power towards deciding what we will be and moving ourselves in the direction of that goal.

What have we felt, just on our own, through eating? For me, I've felt, within my physical self the difference between eating pancakes with syrup for breakfast and scrambled eggs with sausages. Or when I've drank coffee all day forgetting water and food. I even know what my tummy feels like after a night of heavy drinking. I know what clarity comes through fasting. After the hunger subsides. And I realize if I stop binging on ice cream each night before bed and instead do some jumping jacks my body can and will change. Even to the point that I no longer desire the ice cream. But want the work out. I think we can all agree we know from our own experience that our tummies will respond in predictable and certain ways to what we give them to eat.

Okay. What about how our tummies respond to experiences? Have you ever lost your appetite, but not from the flu? Like, perhaps, from being in love… Has your stomach every been in knots over a situation? We can prove for ourselves our digestive systems not only respond to foods but to different circumstances as well.

The interesting and exciting thing is there is now much research that explains and supports what we already know intrinsically if not cognitively. We know our gut is filled with neurotransmitters and is constantly sending signals and receiving signals, in other words, it's talking! All that communication without our overt promptings. We know that the enteric nervous system can be cut off from the brain and carry on without a hitch. That's kinda crazy. Every other system in the body requires the brain. The smooth muscle fibers surrounding our digestive system respond to emotional stimuli. Scientists can trace nerve communications from the gut to the places in the brain that are responsible for morality, emotions, self-awareness, fear, memory, and motivation.

What does all this mean?

I think it means that as Christians, and people seeking a wholeness, that we must not only renew our minds and recover our hearts but also restore our guts.

When an individual has been brought up in an environment of sexual abuse, as I was, the digestive system is essentially trained to operate by darkness. Its operations are perverted. It's not functioning as it was designed to on a daily basis. Our stomachs digest, not only food but our experiences as well. There's a dual functioning. One is visceral. One is invisible. The visceral can give clues to what needs to happen in the invisible. My digestive system was built to process food. If I drink a cup of poison, maybe my body will be able to filter it out and deal with it, but there's gonna be some damage done. Maybe some permanent. Some repairs will be necessary. God's Word tells us we are made for His pleasure and to glorify Him. When we are about this business we are optimally performing. When we are asked (or subject ourselves to) to digest or process poisonous circumstances, like sexual (or any type) abuse, maybe we are able to filter it out and deal with it, but damages occur. Sometimes permanent. But we serve a Great and Mighty God who uses His Might to save! [Thank and praise Him] Because of Him, we may retrain the miles of intestines that have been subjected to sexual trauma and have been desperately working to bring the body back to balance even though the onslaughts just keep coming. Those bowels, from sexual abuse, have received some mortal wounds, then been asked, commanded even, to perform as though everything is hunky dory. "Not cool" says the belly. But as G.I. Joe taught us 'knowing is half the battle' we have an opportunity to make a change.

I want to take a moment and give my belly some hugs, some loves, some accolades. I want to ask my belly what do you need to feel the love? What can I do to help you recover from the subjection to trauma and extreme chronic stress it produces? Then I want to listen...

CHOCOLATE!

Haha. Right! It isn't named theobrama (food of the gods) for naught. Good quality, dark chocolate has some perks. Look into it.

Is your tummy trying to speak to you? Will you listen?

My tummy just said:

'To love me is to take good care of me. Thank you for listening. For offering a chance to speak. I need acceptance. And the chance to feel slow, be slow. Space to feel things that aren't socially acceptable. A safe place to be still.'

To make a fresh start for the tummy, the somatic portion of this handbook takes a great deal of time, energy and intention towards the tummy. It's a beginning place. To heal our guts, it will take a bit of hard work and determination up front. Like the other positive habits, we've trained into our lives, soon, it will feel natural to take appropriate, intentional care of the belly.

What has been helpful for me will not necessarily be the same needs you experience. It's important to learn to be discerning. This learning to discern is little more than focused and intentional listening. Give ourselves safe places to be still, hear what the Holy Spirit would speak to us without judgement against our self. Soon, we will be able to hear Him even in a crowd.

Every single person has got some junk to deal with. The difference for us who've come through long term abuse or a traumatic experience is many times the damages create life dominating behaviors and we cannot pretend everything is okay and function well enough to fool society at large; who all seem to me to be walking around in carefully constructed lies. That's kinda jacked up to say. I know it's gonna piss some people off. Especially those who've grown to believe their own lies. This isn't about that though. It's about taking personal responsibility, before God, with His help and guidance and learning to walk out of the darkness, where we do not know what makes us stumble, and begin walking in The Light of His Presence. Where anything is possible!

For me, God's Word has been most helpful. It builds! What it cuts out of my life is exactly like what our bodies digest and process out. It's smelly, useless and just needs to be flushed away. Everything I do I want to filter through His Word. I might think I hear Him speak, if I can't find a verse to back up what I've heard I want to go back and listen some more. It's a practice and a living relationship. Miscommunications happen constantly for people trying to share their lives face to face constantly. Some miscommunications with The Living, Holy, and Unseen God should not be surprising.

The perfect example, one all of us can easily understand I think, is when we read in the Bible no sex outside of marriage. So, so, so easy to believe our circumstance is different and the one exception because no two people, ever, in the history of the world and lovers and marriage have loved and felt as we do. Not to rain on anyone's parade but that's exactly what we all say. The marriage bed is the only safe place for a man and a woman to express their love physically. Inside the parameters of a lifetime, blood covenant (when the hymen breaks) commitment. Always and only. Yet, our emotions, insecurities, desires for power will lead us to believe an exception exists. It does not. So weird right. Sex is dynamite, only more powerful. We need handling instructions. When I begin to believe it's okay for me to step outside the boundaries set up by God for safe sex, time to go back to His Word, believe it and apply it. That's the method for finding the right path for my life and all the treasures God has set up, just for me, all along the way. The same can be true for you. And will be, if you choose Him.

Towards the restoration of my guts, my first move is to make sure I'm applying God's Word and talking to Him. Secondly, it's imperative I begin with harmless and gentle touch of my abdomen. The goal is to reset the muscle memory and give release and movement to the strong emotional attachments that have been trained into the enteric nervous system. This is best accomplished within the safety of a truly loving same-sex friendship or a trusted marriage partner. It may also be accomplished with a skilled body worker. A guide and sequence are set forth in the second part of this handbook as a place to begin.

Because the physical is intimately tied to the spiritual, what we eat matters to our healing on all the levels. Emotional, physical, spiritual, and mental.

During the writing of this chapter, at the beginning, I was sitting down with a gallon of ice cream and eating almost the whole thing. Stopping only because I became embarrassed my husband would see how much I'd consumed. Maybe I really didn't have the power to choose yoga or an apple, but I could pray! I could ask God to change me; to bless the ice cream and not allow it to harm me. I asked Him to change my desires. And He did! I still have some work towards resisting. A big help is I don't buy a gallon just a pint. And only during my menstruation cycle. I believe I wills top that too. Chiefly because I do not serve a God who's end result is rules. Restrictions. Setting Him up as a babysitter and punisher. No! His end goad is love. Soon, I won't need to make rules for myself. I will simply do what's most loving towards myself. How many of us understand we may destroy our bodies, emotions, mental capacity and spiritual effectiveness with food? But I don't want to do that. I want to do what's most loving. Because I've believed Him, He says I'm loved. His love becomes my love. Besides phasing out ice cream I'm adding options into my diet that are good for my gut. Like leafy greens. Which my rabbit has taught me to enjoy eating plain by the handful. The leafy greens don't seem appealing, yet, once eaten I feel satisfied. Can you imagine feeling satisfied? Furthermore, my belly feels good. I have energy and no regrets. I'm liking these greens more and more! My stomach also loves the citrus and yogurt. The edible sunshine and live cultures bring light and life to my intestines. My point is, find out what feeds and fuels your body to the point of feeling energetic and awesome!

Another exercise I've been practicing recently is using my thoughts to go into my digestive system. Searching with my mind's eye how they are doing. It's helping me determine how different foods actually make me feel.

Physically, for your gut, it's easy to find aids in nurturing the belly. You simply have to look. Check into breathing exercises, herbal teas and different types of exercise. Then, no matter how many times we fall off the horse, we just get right back on.

Matthew 9:36

> *When He saw the crowds, He had compassion on them, because they were harassed and helpless, like sheep without a shepherd.*

Jesus. Completely man and completely God. He left His throne in heaven to come dwell among us and show us The Way to His Father. He was (is) a perfect person. As a perfect person and The Holy God, when He looked upon us, crowds of people, He felt compassion. That word 'compassion' in the Greek New Testament is 'splancnizomai' and means to be moved with pity or compassion. What makes this interesting is that word is made up of the word that is used for intestines, or guts basically. Showing us that in the case of Jesus, our perfect teacher, example, the person (God) we want to emulate, compassion came from His bowels. Deep feelings are somehow stored or even generated down in our bellies. Jesus being perfect, had perfect compassion. We know now, scientifically measurable no less, that the smooth muscles covering our abdomen respond to situations, emotions and stress. Us, not being perfect, is it possible the damage our bodies sustain from stress and trauma affect our capacity to feel and show compassion for others and ourselves? I know that my own ability to experience compassion had been compromised by the almost emotionless reactions I've had in the past to emotional pain I've inflicted on others. I remember, being confused by others reactions to my disrespecting them or hurting them with my words. By God's grace I was interested in these responses and I knew in my will and mind I didn't want to hurt others. But my training warped my understanding and abilities. The humiliations, subjugations, and degradation of being victim to childhood sexual abuse had been woven into the way my intestines worked, my comprehension of how to treat myself and others, and ultimately it shriveled or atrophied my capacity for compassion.

I'm so thankful God is able! Through His Word, knowing it believing it and applying it, He renews our minds, recovers our hearts and restores our digestive systems.

The belly is a responder. It takes what is given and uses that to fuel its thinking and make decisions. As we grow into the ability to take charge of our own bodies, we are able to make decisions regarding what is allowed to enter and influence our enteric nervous system. However, for some of us, the only choice we have is limited to the patterns or habits of thought our brains think. For those cycling through patterns created by abuse and trauma, they are little better than slaves programed and led by degradation into deeper degradation. We have need of nothing short of a Living God willing to break through our darkness with His Light to abolish the effects of abuse and, as crazy or ridiculous, impossible and absurd it may seem, give us the opportunity to be born again by His Spirit and walk ourselves, with His Spirit in our hearts and His hand holding ours, into new life. Victorious life and a health that has no emotional or physical memory of the horrors we've lived through.

Isaiah 61:1,2,3

The Spirit of The Lord God is upon me, because The Lord has anointed me to bring good news to the afflicted; He has sent me to bind up the broken-hearted, to proclaim liberty to captives, and freedom to prisoners; To proclaim the favorable year of The Lord, and the day of vengeance of our God; to comfort all who mourn, to grant those who mourn in Zion, giving them a garland instead of ashes, the oil of gladness instead of mourning, the mantle of praise instead of a spirit of fainting. So, they will be called oaks of righteousness, the planting of the Lord, that he may be glorified.

2 Corinthians 5:17

Therefore, if any man is in Christ, he is a new creature; the old things passed away; behold, new things have come.

2 Corinthians 7:1

> *Therefore, having these promises, beloved, let us cleanse ourselves from all defilement of flesh and spirit, perfecting holiness in the fear of God.*

CHAPTER SIX

Heart

S *ome trust in chariots and some in horses, but we trust in*
The name of The Lord our God Psalm 20:7

Suggested Oils:

Geranium - The oil of love and trust

> "Geranium encourages emotional honesty, love, and
> forgiveness. It fosters receptivity to human love and
> connection. Geranium aids in healing the broken heart."

Peppermint - The oil of a buoyant heart

> "Peppermint brings joy and buoyancy to the heart and
> soul. It invigorates body, mind and spirit, and reminds
> individuals that life can be happy, and they don't have to
> be controlled by fear. When individuals re disheartened,
> they may use peppermint to rediscover the joy of being
> alive."

The Heart Waits

Psalm 27:13-14

I would have despaired
Unless
I had believed
That I would see
The Goodness of The Lord
In the land of the living.
Wait for The Lord;
Be strong
And let
Your heart
Take courage;
Yes, wait for The Lord.

Joshua 1:9

> *Have I not commanded you? Be strong and courageous. Do not*
> *be afraid; do not be discouraged, for The Lord your God will be*
> *with you wherever you go.*

Way back when I was dealing with a load of shame so heavy
it was crippling my ability to stand before people (you know
what I mean? 'stand before people' like be around them and
feel their eyes on me. Feeling so exposed and worthless and
like everyone knows everything about me) I lay on my back,
sort of in prayer. Mostly defeated. But still talking to God.
There was no discernibly visible next step for me. No reason
to get up. But God came near. He descended like a Heavy
Bubble and I felt my heart being crushed, I began to panic.
He whispered, "I'm healing you." I said, "okay". I could
hear in my ears my heart crack, and I felt it. Then the Weight
lifted off. I can't explain what happened. How I heard God.
How I heard my heart crack. What exactly did he do? I don't

know. None the less, I. Believe. Him. He healed something. What and how?

When meditating on this chapter, prior to writing, wanting to hear God and what he would want to say to us girls who've been violated... Well, something weird happened. Through a bizarre series of events I ended up getting my hair cut by a family member. I wanted shoulder length long layers. What I got was shorn. My hair was cut above my ears. It's interesting because I know in the past, I would have believed the family members involved in reassuring me this individual was good at cutting hair and watching me sit down to have my hair butchered, were sabotaging me on purpose. My past belief patterns through abuse training would have taken this event as further proof that no one loves me, I'm worthless. This unfortunate, accidental, misunderstanding could have worked up a family rift. And my heart would have been taken. I would have lost heart for a time. Despairing of being loved or believing that I would ever find love would have drained the courage right out of me.

Those old beliefs. That training from abuse. It waits for an opportunity to strike. It may be dormant in myself somewhere for a time. However, as soon as a situation happens that could be misconstrued, it perks up and comes back with the full force of ugly feelings, like a tidal wave, to devastate my life and take out my heart.

Circumstances. Interactions with others. Perceived motives. Believing half-truths and lies. Little things, big things happen every day for each of us in the normal course of living life that may instigate our hearts being taken. When we are already operating under a load of affliction that is deeply and intimately rooted and intertwined in our hearts and identities, situations that might be minor speed bumps for non-violated, non-traumatized, non-abused individuals, could be like slamming into a granite wall at 60 mph for us. Stops us in our tracks. Pulls a pall of darkness over our eyes and effectively shuts down the heart by despair. Hopelessness.

Okay. Anybody know what I'm talking about?

1 Peter 5:8

> *Be alert and of sober mind. Your enemy the devil prowls around like a roaring lion looking for someone to devour.*

Luke 21:36

> *Be always on watch, and pray that you may be able to escape all that is about to happen, and that you may be able to stand before the Son of men.*

Your heart has value! Our Heavenly Father is after your heart. Because He adores you. He is interested in your best, highest and most joyful life possible. He wants you. All of you. Every place within yourself you want to hide from His sight, He already knows about. He knows about it and He is ready and able and willing to love those bruised and broken places til they come back to life or if they need to be smudged out of existence His love can do that too.

In our hearts, we must know God is on our side. Fighting for us.

Isaiah 35:4

> *Say to those with fearful hearts, 'Be strong, do not fear; your God will come, he will come with vengeance; with divine retribution He will come to save you.'*

We've got to BELIEVE HIM.

Matthew 13:58

> *And He did not do many miracles because of their lack of faith.*

Hebrews 11:6

And without faith it is impossible to please God, because anyone who comes to Him must believe that He exists and that He rewards those who earnestly seek Him.

We need hope there's a reason to find wholeness. If life is just gonna keep on sucking, I'm out. Lemme just self-medicate. I feel that. But I have hope God has something good for me, reserved just for me, in this life. Where I'm respected as a valuable individual. Where I have beautiful, loving relationships. A place where I have a healthy body and something to contribute, I'm excited about. I believe God knew (that's what set me on His path) and knows (what keeps me on His path) the way out of the crap show into the Big show. I just follow Him. Blind faith? I mean, it's not blind because I know his character, He is good. But Sometimes, I can't see where the path He's leading me on is going. But I'm with Him. That makes it all peace. In truth, we might, think apart from God we are ordering our own steps and guiding ourselves on a path that takes us where we want to go. That's all faith too. Faith in self. I choose faith in God, The One who sees not only this step of the journey, but all the way through to the final step. He is The Creator of the universe, The Almighty. Heck ~ to ~ the ~ yee ~ ya ~ yuh.

The Beginning <u>and</u> End. The True and Faithful One. Doesn't your heart just long for The True and Faithful One? Like, when I've behaved so badly, hurt myself and those around me. Feeling like scum and washed up yucky stuff. He is still True and Faithful. He won't be agreeing with my behavior. But He won't be judging me either. Or snickering behind my back. Or blowing smoke up my bung-holio. He's a loving Father. He is there for me. Always. It's a priceless association I'm blessed with. And He is the One who seeks me with kindness and love, even laying down the life of His only begotten Son to make a way to be in relationship with me. I don't know why. I think, because He made us. Because

He is my True Father. Because I know, for my son, what wouldn't I do? To reach him if he needed me. I would do all. Have we any remembrance of true love. The total insanity of it? There's no rhyme nor reason—just perfect harmony that is willing to go ballistic to get to reach it's goal. I'm into that kind of thing. The chaos of abuse and the fake love, I can leave behind and never think of again.

Psalm 16:11

> *Thou wilt make known to me the path of life; In Thy Presence is fulness of joy; In Thy right hand there are pleasures forevermore.*

Jeremiah 29:11

> *"For I know the plans I have for you," declares The Lord. "Plans to prosper you and not to harm you, plans to give you hope and a future."*

Psalm 91:3-4

> *For it is He who delivers you from the snare of the trapper, and from the deadly pestilence. He will cover you with His pinions, and under His wings you may seek refuge; His faithfulness is a shield and bulwark.*

Jeremiah 31:3

> *The Lord appeared to us in the past saying: 'I have loved you with and everlasting love; I have drawn you with unfailing kindness.'*

Zephaniah 3:17

> *The Lord your God is with you. The Mighty Warrior who saves. He will take great delight in you; in His love He will no longer rebuke you, but will rejoice over you with singing.*

John 15: 7-11

If you remain in me and my words remain in you, ask whatever you wish, and it will be done for you. This is to my Fathers glory, that you bear much fruit, showing yourselves to be my disciples.

As The Father has loved me, so have I loved you. Now remain in my love. If you keep my commands, you will remain in my love, just as I have kept my Father's commands and remain in His love. I have told you this so that my joy may be in you and that your joy may be complete.

He has plans for us. Godly plans. We get to participate. What's your dream? Do you dare to dream it? And chase it?

Psalm 37:4

Take delight in The Lord, and He will give you the desires of your heart.

Too good to be true?

Psalm 89:14

Righteousness and justice are the foundation of Thy throne; Loving-kindness and truth go before Thee.

I want justice! I want righteousness! And I believe God is constantly giving me lovingkindness and truth. My heart operates and rests in this. When I find something, someone, some situation is disturbing this peace, I go back to God immediately. In His Word. Asking. Trusting. Believing. He has made my heart free.

John 8:36

So if the Son sets you free, you will be free indeed.

Will You make the choice today to allow your heart to take courage? Allow your heart to hope and believe in The Almighty? The ball is in your court.

Having a courageous heart makes us able and willing to dare to dream! Further to pursue the goal!

CHAPTER SEVEN

Faith Healing? Yes Please!

T *hey are brought to their knees and fall, but we rise up*
and stand firm
Psalm 20:8

Suggested Oils:

Cilantro - The oil of releasing control

> "It is helpful in lightening one's load through the release
> of issues buried in the body, heart, and soul. Cilantro lib-
> erates the soul from heavy burdens, enabling the individ-
> ual to live light and free."

Arborvitae - The oil of divine grace

> "Arborvitae assists individuals who believe or act like all
> progress must be made through struggle and solitary ef-
> fort. Arborvitae is also a grounding oil that teaches Di-
> vinity is all around. God's grace can be felt and experi-
> enced here on earth; it is not distant or separate. Arborvi-

tae's Latin name means 'to sacrifice'. This oil invites individuals to sacrifice their personal will and ambitions for a far more fulfilling way of living."

God's Word is a love letter to us explaining His intentions towards us and the relationship we may enjoy, if we will.

We are a skeptical people. Well versed in doubt. With good reason. Without fail every. single. person. we've ever known has let us down. Even ourselves. Difficult to conceive a Big Man in the sky who has not and will not let us down. Starving children. Slaughtered hearts everywhere. Animals degraded. Natural disasters. All seems like loud, valid proof that there is no benevolence up in the heavenlies.

Faith is about seeing with our hearts. Faith comes by hearing. We require True Words to build our belief on. God understands this. In His infinite kindness He has given to us His Word! Yet, still left enough space for plausible deniability, if we wouldn't receive Him, believe Him, He takes a step back. He has given us dominion on this planet. Check Genesis. We, not God, are responsible for every single act and reaction contrary to love and life and light that happens on this earth. Our own sin has brought about destruction, decay and the ongoing cumulative effects we see daily through the avenues of disease, poverty, and even the natural disruptions. We can be duped into believing our actions are small enough not to matter! But we blame Him. Like a good father, He takes up responsibility on our behalf and provides an out. Whatever's been done to us, whatever we've done to ourselves or others, He has a way out back to wholeness. And yes, YES, He wants to take you, you, Dear, Darling Reader, Precious in His sight you are. You are. Just as you are. Prized by Him. Treasured. You are cherished. He would guide and carry you into your ideal life.

Mark 9:23-24

> *And Jesus said to him, 'if you can!' All things are possible to him who believes. Immediately the boy's father cried out and began saying, 'I do believe; help my unbelief.'*

This is a story of a father seeking healing for his son from Jesus. If you are a parent, you can imagine how high the stakes are. The daddy of this child makes a choice in an instant—to believe. Next moment his own doubt shows itself. His response to that is an example of perfectly executed faith. He exclaims, 'Help my unbelief.' He asks The Giver of all life for help. He doesn't try to hide his doubt or manufacture it on his own. He asks. Knowing he cannot believe on his own that Jesus can or will, or both, heal his boy. He wanted to believe. Had some reason to believe. But when it came to his own situation, was it too risky? Too good to be true? Only he and God know. Evidently it doesn't matter because it is written, the boy was healed that day!

To really believe Jesus, we've got to walk with Him. Complete belief in all He is, is impossible. Chiefly because none of us are capable of completely seeing Him. (I John 3:2). It takes time to walk in consistent, unwavering faith. Like learning to love and trust a life partner. You believe they like you; you take a step. They continue to prove worthy, you continue to move forward. That metaphor begins to break down quickly... Our Father in heaven remembers we are dust (Psalm 103:14) He has given us reassurance in His Word that He wants to heal us. Not us. Me. You. The individual. Crazy as it may present itself to be at first.

Here's some building blocks.

Exodus 15:26

> *He said, 'if you listen carefully to The Lord your God and do what is right in His eyes, if you pay attention to His commands*

and keep all His decrees, I will not bring on you any of the diseases I brought on the Egyptians. For I am The Lord, who heals you.'

At first glance, and because of our training in skepticism, it's like

"Oh. Okay. If I do what you say you won't make me sick. How about sayonara, sucker!"

I get that. But here's what I now know. My Loving Heavenly Father is holding out the path of life for me in His hand, along with the power to walk it and achieve my best life. Plus, joy and love and healing and wholeness all along the way. Following Him naturally leads to the best imaginable for the individual. Better, really, than what we may imagine in our finite minds because we have the Infinite Mind working on our behalf. Further, He will supernaturally protect us from what is overtaking the world. (Psalm 91:7) However, if we refuse Him and go our own way, He permits it. He doesn't have to. He could be the heavenly Dictator instead of Father. If He wanted. He doesn't He allows us to walk into all kinds of disaster. Just as the natural outcome of walking with Him is life and peace. Choosing to walk our own way naturally leads to a diminished life. We think we know the best way for ourself. We've been taught to believe this. To admire and strive for independence. But it's simply not the truth. Neither is it the real desire of our hearts. We were created to crave and function best within the parameters of loving interdependence. With God as our head. So, what He's saying in Exodus 15:26 isn't "I'm the Boss Hog, bow to me or be made sick." Instead, He's saying "let me, please take care of you." We are taught to feel shame at our need to be cared for. That's a trap, don't believe it. God wants your best for you. He wants to heal you. He wants to be with you.

In Exodus 15:26 He names Himself Jehovah Rapha. The God who heals you. He has chosen to make Himself available to you for this purpose and He is able. What God has chosen to be for us, no one has the right to take away. Hebrews 13:8 tells us He is the same yesterday, today, forever. He is The God who healed the Israelites, He is The God who wants to heal you. He will be the God who heals those who come after us.

Doubt:

1. To be uncertain about: consider questionable or unlikely; hesitate to believe.

Romans 8:32

He who did not spare His own Son, but gave Him up for us all how will he not also, along with Him, graciously give us all things.

The most ridiculous notion of all. God loves me. He loves even me. Dare I believe this?

What if it's a ruse and I'm duped again. I can't be duped again. But I can't stay the same.

Proverbs 4: 20-22

My son, attend to my words; incline thine ear unto my sayings. Let them not depart from thine eyes; keep them in the midst of thine heart. For they are life unto those that find them, and health to all their flesh.

A dwelling place where healing is in the air. That's the atmosphere scripture creates for us.

There was a time when I was assaulted by shame, too many times a day to count. This attack was like getting hit on the head with a rubber mallet. Made my brain ring. I'd be in the middle of some activity and it would blast me! Suddenly, I'd become hyper self-conscious, the world around me would be swimming, and all I could feel in my physical self was disgust. At the time, I didn't know how to handle these attacks. Particularly because they'd been occurring since grade school. The first time I remember this happening was second grade. As a child I would disappear within myself to hide and get away from this feeling. As an adolescent I would eat for an instant sensuous and chemical change. As an adult, a cycle of eating, spending, bad relationships, and intoxicants was the antidote. These activities were a desperate attempt to hide and mask the feelings of loathing and hating myself. I believed the feelings and I believed what being sexually abused taught me to think. Basically, that I was perversely foul. There is a demonic influence in there. Wherever children are being abused or women of any age (or men) are being forced into sexual activity, evil is present.

This sudden onset, at any given moment, of shame taking over my brain and feelings was disruptive (to say the least), as you can imagine or may know from experience. It's not easy to function under duress. Living with and learning to overcome sexual abuse is war. Nothing short of covert operations launching hostile blitz attacks in plain sight. I do not have the resources within my personal self to combat this type of aggression. None of us do. But! We have an Advocate! A Victorious King who dresses for battle in a robe that has been dipped in the blood of His enemies (Rev 19:13). He is The One who has the power to throw down our foe of shame invigorated by malicious unseen forces.

The best and most effective way to access His help is by getting a scripture and whipping it out any tie the attack comes. I used Romans 8: 1,2 for like, a year, against the enemy. Yeah. Sometimes it takes a minute to make the onslaught stop for good. The scripture works immediately. Soon as my mind would begin to recite this verse the effects of the shame hammer began to subside. But they came back. Again and again until I was so quick at whipping out my spiritual sword (God's Word: Check Ephesians 6:17) that the shame attack didn't have a chance to interrupt my peace. Then. One day. I realized; this tactic was no longer being employed against me. Keeping myself close to God's Word healed my shame issue and won the battle for good and all. These types of attacks no longer take place in my life.

A problematic effect left for me, from the tidal wave of destruction sexual abuse creates, was a splintered personality. This splintering was caused by those strikes that used my own feelings and thoughts against me on the platform abuse provides. In other words, I've lost time. I have never been diagnosed with any type of dissociative personality disorder but I do know I've 'woken up' in the middle of conversations and had no idea what was going on. I know I've taken one sip of whiskey and blacked out. Just one sip and then have no recollection of the rest of the night. I was on no other drugs, prescription, recreational or otherwise. Completely sober except for one sip. Blacking out comes easy for me. It used to. I don't mess with those alcoholic spirits anymore. Too volatile. Too risky. I've hurt people I love with my words under the influence. My point is, the act of retreating so far within myself that I have no idea what was even making me still functional and not in a coma, that defense mechanism I began practicing in early childhood to protect myself from circumstances so scary I simply vanished—even that debilitating function that I had no control over and didn't even realize was operating until well into my thirties. God knew. Through my association with Him and creating a habitat for myself with His Word, He's proved Himself True and Faithful over and over and over again. But to me personally. He's just cleared that away. I no longer lose time. He did that for me. No medication. No long gross talks with therapists. Just me and Him. Walking together. Living life. He will do the same for you. Personally. In a unique way fitted perfectly to you.

Romans 8:1,2

There is therefore now no condemnation for those who are in Christ Jesus. For the law of The Spirit of life in Christ Jesus has set you free from the law of sin and death.

I've taken mortal wounds to my soul. But because of Jesus I get to live. And not just scrape by dragging my poor beat up self around. No way Jose! I get to thrive! Check me out!

Quick Chat

Evil influences. What am I talking about? Demons? Possession? Exorcism? Yes and no.

2 Pitfalls

1. Giving the enemy too much attention and credit

2. Ignoring or denying the enemies ability

Enemy = Satan. Yes. Him. He is real.

Remember; God created the enemy and has a plan to terminate his activity. Check John 1:3, Colossians 1:16-17 / Revelation 17-19

God is bigger. God is badder. God will prevail.

1 John 4:4

You, dear children are from God and have overcome them, because The One who is in you is greater than the one who is in the world.

1 John 5: 4-5

> *For everyone born of God overcomes the world. This is the victory that has overcome the world, even our faith. Who is it that overcomes the world? Only the one who believes that Jesus is The Son of God.*

Defense: As ever, stay in God's Word. Read it aloud if you feel surrounded. That will clear the air. Speak aloud to Jesus, using His Name, it is above every Name and evil personalities won't stick around to listen.

1 Timothy 4:7

> *Have nothing to do with irreverent, silly myths. Rather train yourself for godliness.*

The best way to deal with evil is to discipline yourself with God's Word. For those of us who've accepted Jesus as our Savior, invited Him to live inside our heart and to be born again by His Spirit, we are never alone. He is always with us. His Presence and learning to skillfully wield His Word is our first and best line of defense. Second, sometimes we need back-up. It is crucial for each of us to have someone we can call on to help us pray. A prayer partner, mentor, spiritual mother; if you do not have a person before whom you may be completely transparent and call on anytime for help and comfort, ask God to send you someone. Many times, I've had to call in the 'big guns. Meaning reach out to prayer partners and/or spiritual mentors to pray with me and for me.

Matthew 18: 19,20

> *Again, truly I tell you that if two of you on earth agree about anything they ask for it will be done for them by My Father in heaven. For where two or three are gathered in My Name, there am I with them.*

1 John 4:1

Dear friends, do not believe every spirit, but test the spirits to see whether they are from God, because many false prophets have gone out into the world.

The enemy of our souls is not playing fair. He has no interest in civilized warfare. He will attack the wounded guaranteed. He will bait and switch. He comes only to steal God's Word away from you. Kill your hope and destroy your life.

John 10:10

The thief comes only to steal, kill and destroy; I have come that they may have life, and have it to the full.

The prescription for dealing with evil spirits is go to God's Word as soon as the influence is suspected or detected. Call for back-up. Pray continually. Finally, stand your ground.

Ephesians 6:10-18. Put on the full armor of God. And having done all stand.

Matthew 7:7-11

Ask. Seek. Knock.

Our heavenly Father is interested in us. He cares about the details of our lives. He wants to communicate with us. He encourages us to ask. Seek. Knock. He tells us we will receive if we do.

Luke 18:1-8 That persistent widow.

Don't stop asking, seeking, and knocking until you get what you want or through prayer come to understand you want something else.

I cannot say why God even cares about me. Except I know He does. My little boy asks me why I love him sometimes. I don't have a sufficient answer for that either. It isn't because he's good or easy or adds something valuable to my life. Although that's true it's also true he's naughty sometimes, is definitely far and away the most challenging and difficult 'work' I've ever done. Sometimes, realistically, he's terribly inconvenient. Like first thing in the morning before I've had my coffee and he vomit all over the bed, then poops through his diaper. Then after all that's cleaned up and I finally have a cup of hot coffee he wants to climb into my lap and somehow knocks my cup just right so it flips up into the air and lands on my head spilling hot coffee all down me. Oh yeah. True story. I don't even care. I just love him. Regardless. Condition less. He's mine. Maybe God feels the same about us.

Condition-less isn't to say we have no role of participation in this thing. He is no push-over, doormat, meal ticket or sugar daddy. He's a real person. A real person who is also God. Salvation is free, all His gifts are free. It's like with my husband, whatever he has is mine, as long as I am respecting and loving him only. That's appropriate. It's beautiful. It's all the wonderful colors of the rainbow. It's free, yet it costs me my entire life as well. The same is true with The Living God, the most Passionate Person of all. He will want nothing less than all of you. As He has demonstrated He gives nothing less than His all. And that's a good trade.

Isaiah 30: 18

Yet the Lord longs to be gracious to you; therefore he will rise up to show you compassion. For The Lord is a God of justice. Blessed are all who wait on Him.

Look to The Lord. That is where your help comes from...

PART 2

The Sequences

*L*ord, give victory to The King! Answer us when we call.

Psalm 20:9

1. Who to practice with?

2. Goals of sessions

3. Essential Oils: Why and how?

4. Directing the breath

5. Forehead Pull/Foot Rub

6. Set up your space

7. What this is and is not

8. Going into Session

1. It Takes Two

When I was going through massage therapy school my question was always "How can I do this myself?" My instructor always replied "You can't."

Inherent in these sequences is a necessity to trust another with our bodies and emotions. It's all a learning process.

To my way of thinking, the very best person to work with is a trusted same-sex bestie. Your ride or die. To have the gift of a safe relationship where you may be all the worst aspects of yourself without fear of being rejected or of having the ugly stuff thrown back in your face, this gift if priceless. I hope you have such a one.

A loving, supportive spouse could be an excellent partner in this work. Sometimes, memories could surface or feelings that have potential to create a speed bump in a marriage relationship. I don't hide things from my husband, but I am thoughtful (strategic) about how, what and when I speak to him of the abuse and fallout thereof from my past. In order to assist me in my healing journey, he would need to forget himself, his feelings, his attachment to the ideas he has of who I am. Who I am now, took a lot of years of work and mistakes, big ones, have been made? Those things have nothing to do with him, if he had to hear and know all the gory details that sometimes come out during a session, how is he going to respond? The marriage relationship isn't necessarily a therapeutic relationship for trauma. Be certain this is something your relationship can handle. If you guys agree this is safe, go for it. A spouse is my second choice.

The third option is finding a massage therapist. A good therapist will ask you at the beginning of what your needs are and this is when you present what it is you want to achieve. Allow the therapist to see the sequences. This work is definitely not for every massage therapist out there. It may take a minute to find one who is willing and has the ability to assist you. Don't give up!

2. Goals of Practice

A. The body memory factor addressed, retrained.

B. Resurrecting the abdomen.

C. Reconnecting the reproductive system with pleasure.

3. Essential Oils: Why and how?

This wheezing rasping sound was always showing up from the bottom of my lungs once we were finished practicing the act of marriage. It was disconcerting to both of us. You know the feeling? Like when something seems to be going wrong inside your body but you have no idea what... What happens next? The flood of 'what if's' associated with the unknown and all the panic and fear that wants to come too!

My husband and I were discussing it and he said why not use one of your oils. I was like 'oh yeah. Duh!'

So, I fetched the respiratory blend from my oils shelf and we rubbed that over my hearts and lungs. My husband prayed for me and that was that. We forgot about it. Next thing we know, sometime later, we noticed. "Hey, the wheezing is gone." We both laughed and said, "Cool" and moved on.

The circumstance does warrant pause. I had a recurring physical situation we both could hear and I felt. One evening we simply and faithfully applied an essential oil, prayed to Jesus, and then forgot about it. Then the physical occurrence disappeared. We applied essential oils and faith. No cumbersome doctor visits. No invasive weird chats with shrinks about why...just a simple act of faith.

This is just one experience in one girl's life of faith and essential oils working. I believe essential oils work. I believe they are a gift from God. I believe they are an important physical companion to prayer. I use them daily for general purposes and specific. I use them on my three-year-old and have since his birth. I use them on my husband, my animals and in the air by diffuser and in our food. With my whole and believing heart I recommend them to you also, for use during your journey through dealing with trauma and further, for use on your journey through life.

The main reason I believe they are super helpful with trauma work is because our olfactory sense is our only sense attached to the limbic system. The limbic system deals with emotions and memory. Each essential oil has different constituents that lend itself to being helpful in specific areas. Areas like grief, confidence, fear—I mean really, you name the area—and there's a specific oil that can be applied with a great likelihood of help. Oils work best as preventatives with regular use, as I understand them. There is vast information out there to help you learn more about different aspects of oils whether you care about how they are harvested or how they were used in Biblical times or even scientific measurements of the vibrational frequency of oils and how they react to prayer. There's so much to learn. When I consider the mountains of information, I recognize my own ignorance. I'm still learning! If you choose to add essential oils to your life, I would be honored to have the opportunity to be of some service to you in this area. You can purchase the essential oils from my website at (gutsandvictory.com). Or if you're interested in becoming a member for wholesale privileges please email me at (cora@gutsandvictory.com) and I will do my utmost to be helpful.

The term 'essential' applied to oils means the oils that come from the plant are essential to that plant's life. These oils aren't essential to your healing journey. I do believe they may serve you as a major help and comfort.

Another thing I need to say is I'm not a medical doctor. I am not authorized or trained to advise anyone in matters that pertain to their physical health. I am a voice and a witness of what has worked for me. I am a wellness advocate associated with a certain oils company but I am what might be called a brick in the wall. I have not worked to become an oils sales person. I have worked to know God and share with you what He has done in my life. Sure, I want my oils business to grow. But it will never be the main thing I have to say to you. If you want to join me, I want you too! If not, I'm psyched to have the chance to share with you. I think that completes my pitch and disclaimers and I hope it's satisfactory.

How to Use:

I have suggested specific oils for each chapter dealing with different subjects that have been related to my experience with trauma as well as specific oils for each of the three massage sessions laid out. I have chosen these sometimes intuitively and sometimes based on information I have read out of different essential oil companion books. The oils I have chosen are meant to be used topically and aromatically. If you choose to ingest the oils it is important to be well informed and, in some cases, check with your doctor.

For aromatic use it's really helpful to have a diffuser which you can buy from my website, your local health food store, online, and as they are gaining popularity, I've seen them popping up for sale in unexpected places such as department stores.

If you don't have a diffuser you can simply place a drop of oil in the palm of your hand, rub your hands together then cup them over your nose and inhale. Ahhh. I'm going to do that now with… hmm. Lavender and peppermint. Peppermint is off the chain powerful guys. Hold on I'll be right back. So, I inhaled the lavender then the peppermint then I felt like rubbing the pep over my lower abdomen and that felt so good I got the aroma-touch blend for my lower back. I've been sitting a long time trying to type all this stuff to you.

For topical use you may apply the oils neat over the area of interest. Be advised some oils may cause skin irritations and need to be mixed with a carrier oil such as olive oil or coconut oil. Mostly I learn my oils through trial and error. When in doubt us a carrier oil. Start slow and slow down. Like I said there's tons of information about oils everywhere. I cannot possibly cover everything here and besides we have other work to do.

4. Breath work

Pnuema is the word in the Greek New Testament that is used for Holy Spirit. Part of that definition means 'breath'. In Genesis God brings the thing he made of clay to look like a man, to life, by breathing into him. If we stop breathing, we cease to live. Mostly we take all that for granted and pay little attention to our breathing. Allowing oxygen into our bodies and cognitively directing it to a certain place, such as ankles, with healing intentions will make a big difference for us in our whole lives and for this massage sequence. Here are a couple of exercises I copied directly from a book I like called *The Woman's Belly Book*. If you already have breathing exercises you use and like, implement those. Otherwise, here is an easy way to begin...

Directing the Breath[3]

1. Sit or lie comfortable. Allow your breath to deepen into your belly, and enter into the Centering Breath.

2. As you breathe, notice the images and sensations occurring within your belly. See and feel the life energy focused within your belly center growing brighter and stronger with each breath.

3. Breathing in through your hara[4], send the breath from your hara to any area in your body that needs warmth, energy, attention, or healing, and breathe out through that place. (As attention and energy return to a site that's been numb or injured, the sensations that accompany the increased awareness may be a bit uncomfortable. Go slowly, with the intention to witness rather than resist sensation. Your breath and your compassionate awareness will encourage the process of healing.)

4. Closing your eyes, take a few moments to experience the images and sensations occurring in the area through which the breath is flowing.

5. Gradually return your awareness to this time and place.

Centering Breath

1. Set the stage for this deep abdominal breathing by giving yourself room to breathe. Adjust your clothes and your posture to allow your belly to move out and in easily with your

---

[3] From The Woman's Belly Book: Finding Your True Center for More Energy, Confidence, and Pleasure by Lisa Sarasohn. (Page 206)

[4] The Japanese use a single word, hara, to name the belly both as a physical region of your body and as your connection to Source Energy. Your hara extends from the base of your ribs to the upper margin of your pubic bone, deepening inward to your spine. Within this region, a few inches below your navel, is your belly center. (Page 111)

breath. Unhitch your waistband, loosen your belt, unzip your zipper. Sit or stand comfortable. Adjusting your posture to allow your belly to move freely. Place your palms on your lower abdomen.

2. Notice what's happening underneath your hands. You might already sense a wavelike motion, your belly expanding away from your spine as you inhale and then sinking back toward your spine as you exhale.

3. If you don't see or sense any movement, that's okay. You can jump-start the process by actively pulling your belly in toward your spine as you exhale. Then release the contraction and allow your belly to relax. As it expands naturally—you don't need to push it outward—your belly draws the breath in, beginning the inhalation.

4. Continue, keeping your mouth closed and allowing the breath to move evenly in and out through your nose.

5. Feel the gentle rhythm, allowing your belly to expand and draw the breath in, and then to sink back toward your spine and send the breath out. You might imagine that your belly contains a beautiful balloon. With each inhalation, the balloon fills with breath, and your hands ride with your belly away from your spine. With each exhalation, the balloon empties; your hands ride with your belly back in toward your spine.

6. Continue observing your belly and your breathing for ten or more cycles of breath.

7. Gradually return your attention to your whole body and to the present moment.[5]

---

[5] From The Woman's Belly Book: Finding Your True Center for More Energy, Confidence, and Pleasure by Lisa Sarasohn. (Page 29)

5. Forehead Pull/Foot Rub

The head and the feet are both areas whereby one may succinctly reach the whole body for the purposes of releasing tension, increasing circulation and improving thought processes.

Forehead

The forehead has the *frontalis* muscles. These muscles can crinkle up when we are thinking too hard or holding our breath. The third eye is supposed to be found in the center but just above the eyebrows. This area, some believe can get rather clogged and requires a little help to get the energy flowing again. Also, this point is connected to the pineal gland which is part of the endocrine gland and responsible for the production of melatonin. So that sounds super relaxing! Mainly, it feels good and is certainly relaxing to have another, sort of, wipe away the stress of trauma work from your brow.

This is easy and effective.

Begin with laying your thumbs on the beginning points of the inner eyebrows. Apply a bit of pressure equivalent to the weight of your hands and drag thumbs across the eyebrows following the natural arch of them. Repeat several times. Massage leaves room for improvisation. If it feels natural and necessary move your thumbs up just a tad and do this same motion slightly higher than the eyebrow and following the same arch.

Next, place the pads of your four fingers over the eyebrow and drag up and stop at the hairline. Then once reaching the hairline use those same fingertip pads and sort of flutter feather walk the fingers back down to the eyebrow and repeat. Three times is enough. But you aren't limited by these suggestions.

Finally, hold the head with fingers splayed about the middle or ear level. Thumbs resting in the center of the forehead just above the brow line. Here is a chance to pray over your person, aloud is nice. Do what you do. Maybe you sing a quiet song. Maybe you observe the silence. Repeat a scripture perhaps. After a few moments. Remove your hands. Then proceed with your session be it beginning or ending.

Feet

Your person may be in any position which is comfortable for them or they may be in prone or supine positions for this part of the session.

Focus on one foot at a time.

Begin by holding the ankle with one hand and the heel with the other, supporting the foot from underneath using your thumbs to manipulate the tissues on top with gentle pressing around where your thumbs naturally reach. Giving gentle squeezes to the heel.

Then it is well to continue holding the foot by the heel and taking the other hand and using the knuckles to rub up and down the sole of the foot. Then in circular motions.

Finally, if you have access to a reflexology chart and want to apply pressure to certain areas on the foot to stimulate different parts of the body do that. Now is also a swell time to give some gentle kneading with the thumbs to the sole of the foot and the finger tips on the top of the foot. Remember, on the tops of the feet to use much gentleness for those little bones require it.

6. Set Up Your Space

Creating a safe space and inspired takes just a little thought.

Some ideas for lovely ways to invite intimacy, warmth, and feelings of serenity to your session space are as follows

-Candles

-instrumental music or sounds of nature

-soft blankies

-pillows

-favorite teddy or stuffed friend

-soft lights

-plants and/or flowers

-cozy, comfy clothes

-devices turned off and, in another room,

-no television

-doors locked or area otherwise secured for privacy

Just some ideas. This is your session and your space. Add whatever makes you feel good and take away whatever does not.

7. What this is and is not

This is a practice anyone can do. It takes an open heart and a willingness to be vulnerable. Give yourself patience. Compassion. And room to make a mistake if that's what happens, okay. There isn't really any way to make too big a mistake with loving and gentle touch with pure intentions.

This is not a perfection or professional type deal. This is for you. Make it your own. The work can be heavy it can be sad it can inspire rage or even a negative physical response such as vomiting. Let this practice be surrounded by an attitude of gratitude and high hopes. Knowing, you'll come out the other side with something new. Even though ugly, terrible, horrifying circumstances have given impetus for this work, we (with God's help {Romans 8: 27, 28} It is the will of God to work all things for good in your life!) can still make it beautiful. Powerful. And beneficial. Our attitudes, our reactions are ours to choose. I want to make mine count for good! I want so much for us. It starts within ourselves. Our own healing. Our own attitudes. You know, if God is on our side who can stand against us. We are operating from a field of victory already if we know and love and trust Him. The game is ours to lose. But let's win. Yes!

Also, I am not qualified to write a manual on massage therapy (the things I'm not qualified to do just keep stacking up!) this book is written with the idea that God is the one who heals and He has included us in His plans. He makes us able to help one another. I've worked with many ladies who are believers and have realized that God has made His people peculiar to Him indeed! We simply ask Him and He will give us the healing power in our touch for one another. It sounds so unbelievable. Asking? And believing? What am I nuts? It's been suggested. But, no. I'm not. I just believe God. Still, there is skill in a massage therapists' hands. If you have literally no experience touching another for massage it's super simple to go online to your search engine of choice and look up basic massage strokes. This will give you some knowledge and maybe a bit of confidence to begin. I'm including basic massage strokes below with very basic definitions so that later when I'm laying out a sequence and I suggest a certain type of stroke we may be on the same page about what this means. These are just suggestions. It's a beginning place. The more you practice the more you'll feel at ease and the best part is you'll be working with your pal, so that always makes the work easier.

Effleurage: Long gliding strokes

Petrissage: Kneading

Friction: Warming stoke with more pressure

Tapotement: Percussive stroke

8. Going into Session

The Practitioner:

Pray. Pray. Pray. Pray. And then pray some more. That means get in touch with The Living God. Invite Him. Ask His Spirit to descend like a dove and move like a mighty wind through your session. Praise Him with voice and dance. Do whatever you do and do whatever you can in faith to make yourself realize He is with you. He promises never to leave us or forsake us so factually He is present. He isn't always tangibly present and we don't have the power to force Him to make His Presence felt. Our God values faith. Our goal is to pray and praise Him until we are armed with the knowledge and unwavering conviction, He is with us. Like, in my mind I know He is with me always like on an information level, when I pray heaven down, I *feel* He is with me too. Not necessarily tangibly but in myself, my heart, I'm convinced on a deeper level that He is going before me, hedging me in behind and before and moving around and through all. You know, guys, it takes a bit of time, focus, and work—anything worth having will. We all want the magic wand; it seems so easy and quick. But that's kinda the definition of cheap right?

We've invited God, we know and feel He is with us. Now to approach your subject: your friend, this little girl woman. This individual created by God and who He would have died for were she the only one because that's how amazeballs He IS. She is highly valued. Cherished. Chosen. Lovely all through. We want clean hands and an innocent heart to approach her and touch her. It is good to realize you are given a privilege to lay hands on a child of God. Whatever your faith, this is a child of God. That's something! 7.8 billion peoples on the earth. What's the big deal? Our God knows and loves the individual. He is infinite and loves each of us infinitely. Just believe it and recognize, this small one under your hands was made in God's image and someone has maligned her. We have the awesome privilege of bringing a gift, that touch, from God, delivered through you to her. We can give this to each other. Lets!

Approaching a naked female laying before you covered only by a sheet is a bit like befriending a rabbit. Cover yourself with the quiet that comes from heaven, let it seep into your heart. Let your movements be defined by gentility, and your mind robed in peace. You are in charge of this session, she has allowed you here, if you are comfortable, she will be able to relax and be comfortable to. You will let her know your comfort level by being natural in the room. If, when you enter, you see the sheet is askew you will naturally walk around her and fix the sheet always, always, always honoring the body with modesty and proper covering. No mistakes here, guys, this is a big trust builder. Sometimes if I've been nervous entering the session room and I haven't yet put my hands on the individual I turn my heart and mind to a praise song to Jesus, this takes my mind to something (someone) beautiful and gives me a freedom of movement while the subject is searching me with her spirit to check me out. Maybe next you light a candle or set your oils closer or whatever the business is before you actually lay your hands on the subject. Okay. Stage is set. When your hands first go on the subject lay them down and leave them. For example, session one the subject will be face up. If you place the hands on the abdomen to begin with do not move them for the time it takes for everyone to gain calmness and confidence. There is a communication taking place between your hands and the person's belly. There is a communication that has been taking place between your spirits. Now allow your subjects body to relax under your touch. This can take several minutes but it is important, sometimes essential. If your subject isn't relaxed you will not be able to accomplish much. Once you've felt within yourself the communication line linked, you may begin.

These first moments that begin the session set up the tone for the rest of your time. Let yourself take the time you need to establish a foundation for your session that is built upon trust in one another. Once you establish this what happens during the session can easily be moved through. The sheet slips, you drop the oil, somehow a phone gained access and rings or dings, you accidentally press the wrong muscle, somebody sneezes or other bodily functions occur, whatever. Once the trust is established you have freedom to work.

The Subject:

Pray. Breath. Bring your mind back to what's happening. Stay present. Allow yourself to receive and believe this is coming from God through your session partner.

If at any time you're uncomfortable or don't like something, speak up!

If the session is becoming intense and you feel like stopping, maybe you need to stop maybe you need to push through, you will be the one to decide this. You can always begin again at another time.

These sessions may all be worked with the traditional nakedness under the sheet with the practitioner moving the parts of the sheet to expose the area being focused on as she goes. These sessions may be worked with the person nude but not moving the sheet to expose naked flesh, the work may be done over the sheet. Or a person may remain clothed in comfy stuff like sweats or yoga gear. It's totally up to you and your comfort level. I just always say and think 'naked' because of my massage therapy training.

Pray. Breath. Keep yourself present.

SESSION 1

Goal: Resurrecting the abdomen

Scripture Focus: Psalm 23

Suggested oils:

Bergamot - The oil of self-acceptance

> "Bergamot relieves feelings of despair, self-judgement, and low self-esteem. It supports individuals in need of self-acceptance and self-love. Bergamot invites individuals to see life with more optimism. Bergamot has a cleansing effect on stagnant feelings and limiting belief systems. Because of core beliefs of being bad, unlovable, and not good enough, they seek to hide behind a façade of cheerfulness. They may fear revealing their true thoughts and feelings."

Black Pepper - The oil of unmasking

> "Black Pepper invites individuals to get real by digging deep within the less understood parts f the self. Whether one's true motives and feelings are acknowledged or not, they continue to exist. The more these feelings are pushed down, buried, and repressed, the more they seek to make themselves known. If they are not honestly dealt

with and acknowledged, they will often be expressed through erratic, compulsive, or addictive behaviors. Black Pepper also reignites the soul fire, fueling motivation and high energy, and hastening the healing process."

Ginger - The oil of empowerment

"Ginger powerfully persuades individuals to be fully present and participate in life. Ginger addresses deep patterns of victim mentality, which is evidenced by feelings of powerlessness, believing everything is outside one's control, refusing to take responsibility for life, or blaming life circumstances on other people or outside influences. Victims feel stuck as they decentralize or disown responsibility and blame others for their misfortunes. Ginger empowers individuals in take complete responsibility for their life circumstances."

Grapefruit - The oil of honoring the body

"Grapefruit teaches true respect and appreciation for one's physical body. It supports individuals who struggle to honor their body and are caught in patterns of mistreatment. These forms of abuse may include severe dieting, judging one's body weight or type, and abusing the body through negligent behavior or violence. These acts are often motivated by hate and disgust buried within the psyche, which gets directed toward the physical body. Grapefruit encourages integrity by respecting one's physical needs. This oil assists individuals in listening to their true physical needs and impulses. It also assists them in taking responsibility for what they feel."

Frankincense - The oil of truth

> "Frankincense reveals deceptions and false truths. It invites individuals to let go of lower vibrations, lies, deceptions, and negativity. This oil helps create new perspectives based on light and truth. Frankincense recalls to memory spiritual understanding, gifts, wisdom, and knowledge that the soul brought into the world. It is a powerful cleanser of spiritual darkness. Frankincense assists in pulling the "scales of darkness" from the eyes, the barriers from the mind, and the walls from the heart. Through connecting the soul with its inner light, this oil reveals the truth."

Cypress - The oil of motion and flow

> "Cypress teaches the soul how to let go of the past by moving with the flow of life. This oil is especially indicated for individuals who are mentally or emotionally stuck, stiff, rigid, tense over striving or have perfectionistic tendencies. Cypress encourages individuals to cast aside their worries and let go of control so they can enjoy the thrill that comes from being alive."

For my sessions I would choose an essential oil to use in the diffuser. I took a drop or two of each of these six essential oils and added them to a cup of olive oil. This I used over the abdomen. How much or how little oil to use is entirely up to the individuals practicing. Use whichever essential oils appeal to you. Use all the essential oils suggested or use none or anywhere in between. Your session. Your essential oils. Your choice.

Session Direction

This session is worked with the subject laying on their back or supine position. (This can feel more vulnerable than prone position)

This section may be worked entirely over the sheet if the subject prefers. Or you may pull the sheet down to the hip bones using another smaller piece of fabric to cover the breasts. The mammary glands have been made symbols of sexual desire, been subjected to criticism on their size and the way they look, there are some who argue it is demeaning to the woman to cover them during massage sessions. Whatever. I'm not here to argue that. I'm here to say modesty is a protection. It is better for the purposes of these sessions to keep parts of the body that have been super sexualized covered. It's so good to just relax, exhale, feel safe and not have to prove to the world you can be a big woman and have your breasts exposed during a massage session. It's okay to want the sheet. It's okay to move the sheet. For these purposes let's maintain strict lines of modesty whether it's a felt need or not.

As I sit down to attempt and lay out a step by step map for you who want to use this tool on your journey to wholeness, I'm thinking of Corrie ten Boom who said, "faith sees the invisible, believes the unbelievable and receives the impossible." And Colossians 1: 16,17 "By Him all things were created, both in the heavens and on the earth, visible and invisible, whether thrones or dominions or rulers or authorities—all things have been created by Him and for Him. And he is before all things, and in Him all things hold together." It's a joy to be able to communicate with you and I'm thankful to God. He has given us authority through using His Name, which is above every other name, to pray to Him and move mountains. For this session I wish to ask Jesus to guide me that we may move the mountain of hurt that has taken up residence in the belly. The prolonged stress in response to the tension the whole abdomen has been holding on with and endeavoring to function through because of offense committed against this person. The wholeness sought warrants attention given to the whole person. This includes our guts. Our beautiful. Sweet. Tender bellies need.

> Lord God, guide us into erasing, as writing on a chalk board, the pain in our bellies, reveal the unhealthy habits we've adopted to try and cover the pain and give us courage and passion to, by faith, know You've healed us and changed us and made us able to begin training ourselves for new habits. Healthy and loving habits that nourish our physical bellies that have been slaving away working to digest the poison of sexual violation. We know the spiritual and physical are tied in such a way that we may not observe their separate beginnings and endings. But you, Lord, you see the whole, you see the pieces, and we believe you to mercifully lend us power and attend our session. Thank you, Jesus. Amen.

I'm using the Bergamot and Black Pepper on my hands to begin this session. My person is lying face up as I rub my hands over and above her face that she may inhale the aromas of self-acceptance and unmasking. If she doesn't mind, I have essential oils on my hands I will put the palm of my hand over her third eye and press down with the same pressure I'd use to press against my own eyeball. Then after a moment, sustaining the pressure I will drag my palm to the hair line and lift off my hand then do this twice more to clear the mind.

Now I will move to her left side. Left or right, if it matters, I don't know why, this is just the side I am personally comfortable on.

Both hands have been placed on the belly. Left hand more or less over the belly button. Pause for the introduction of hands to another's body. Now I begin the clockwise circles, fingertips slightly lifted off abdomen while length of fingers and palms are the surface area touching the belly. When ready bring fingertips to rest over point one on illustration 1.A. Let contact with the stomach be made, take your time, bring your attention back and breath. By faith we believe what we speak over the stomach is coming to pass. Believe with your mind, believe with your feelings, and allow your body to become and antenna that receives and transmits the grace of God. Lead your person to repeat after you:

"Thank you, stomach. I give you Infinite Light by the grace of God."

After your person has had a chance to repeat this, without hurry, begin small clockwise circles over the stomach point. Stop. Then move down to point two on figure 1.A. Repeat this process for points 1-9 calling each point by its corresponding organ name. And speaking grace over each point.

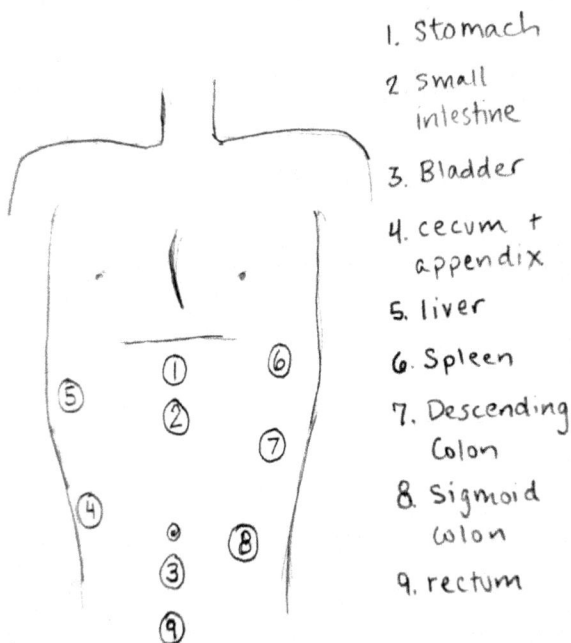

1. Stomach
2. Small intestine
3. Bladder
4. cecum + appendix
5. liver
6. Spleen
7. Descending Colon
8. Sigmoid Colon
9. rectum

Figure 1.A

6

Once that is complete, without losing contact, from point 9 begin your big clockwise circles over the belly again with the fingertips slightly lifted using palms and length of fingers as contact area.

Look to figure 1.B

Repeat the same process for figure 1.A of bringing fingertips to rest approximately over area marked. This is a

---

6 The illustrations i.e. Figure 1.A, Figure 1.B and Figure 1.C were gleaned from Eastern Chinese Medicine

chance to speak to the anxiety, fear, sorrow, and anger that may be hiding in the belly. Call it by name and ask it to leave. Intentionally replacing each bad feeling with glad feelings. The replacement feelings being suggestions. Maybe you guys prefer to replace anger with love. Or sorrow with peace. It's your session!

Example: fingertips resting over point one for **figure 1.B,** therapist may pray:

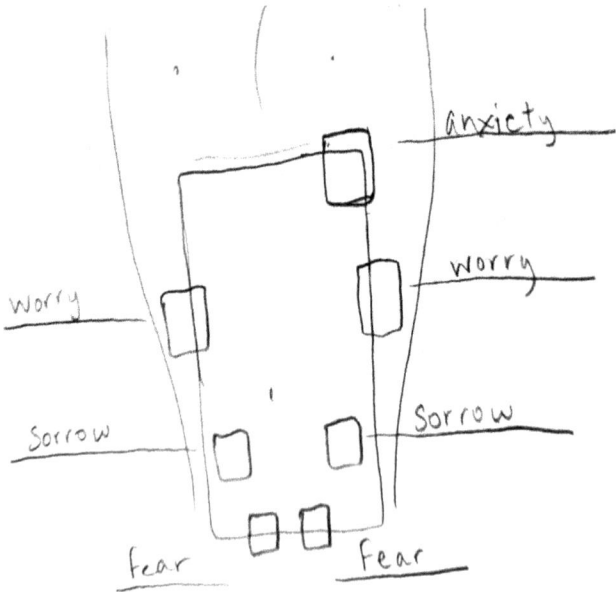

Figure 1.B

In the Name of Jesus, I ask anxiety to leave this girl. You are no longer needed. Thank you. I ask courage to fill up your vacated space to overflowing. That this girl will walk in boldness and beauty. Thank you, Jesus, for your help.

Do this over points 1-7 asking all the worry and fear and sorrow and anger to leave replacing them with fruit of The Spirit or good things like compassion and courage. Once that is complete begin your big circles again.

Now is a good time to take a pause. I would move around the individual adjusting the sheet. Perhaps a drink of water, adjust temperature, check in with your partner see how they are doing if they need any adjustments. After a breather I would take some essential oil, combining a drop each of grapefruit, frankincense and cypress in my palm. Rub it over the abdomen in the clockwise circles. Now moving onto figure 1.C bring the fingertips to rest on point A. This point is about two finger widths below the belly button. Apply just enough pressure that your person knows where your fingertips are resting. It's most comfortable for me to use the pointer, middle and ring fingers of both hands pressing into the point while the thumbs and pinky fingers take flight. Here is the point where we will be speaking thanksgiving to God; forgiveness: from God, from self, for other; and seeking to invigorate and reinforce our personal power. Friends, there is no guide for this. Use your own words. Have your subject use her words. Let out what needs to be let out. And cast out what needs to be cast out. Believe God and receive from Him what He has for you alone.

Finishing this lift, the hands off the belly. Turn your body so you may comfortably lay one whole hand on the chest of your person with the middle finger just resting on point B from figure 1.C. This is a repeating exercise again where it's time to affirm love and wholeness over the physical and spiritual body. Use your own words.

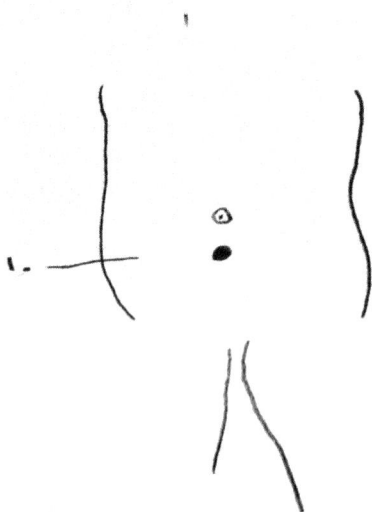

1. Conception Vessel (6)
   chinese medicine

Figure 1.C

For example: I declare in Jesus's Name that I am whole and healed. That I may begin to walk in victory on a new level. I receive power from God to use my voice and determine to speak truth in love. Thank you, Lord. Yes! and Amen!

To finish this session, cover the body again with the sheet. Maybe throw an extra blanket over the body to add comfort and warmth. Move to the head of the individual to proceed with the forehead pull to give comfort, pleasure, a wind down time and a farewell from your hands and heart.

Congratulations you've finished your first session. I would give it a week or two before starting the next. After your session be sure and hydrate, the water will help flush impurities. It's also a good time to break out the old journal and jot down a record of your session. Feelings. Flashes. Movements. Shifts. It has happened that I've worked this session on a person and she has felt nothing. Then later she's noticed changes. It has also happened that I've worked this session and the person felt a great deal of physical pain afterwards that was almost crippling. The pain didn't last, but it showed itself. However, there was nothing changed. How can I explain this? I can't. Our bodies can be mysterious extremely to us. It is well to focus on the fact that there is nothing hidden from God. With this work, the only way out is through. Hold fast your hope and faith and you will not be disappointed finally. And I don't mean when you're dead. Like King David, I expect to see the goodness of The Lord in the land of the living! Psalm 27:13 I hope that this will be your expectation too.

SESSION 2

Goal: The body memory factor addressed and retrained

Scripture Focus: Psalm 91

Suggested Oils:

Cinnamon - The oil of Sexual Harmony

> "Cinnamon dispels fear of rejection and nurtures healthy sexuality. It rekindles sexual energies when there has been repression, trauma or abuse. Cinnamon invites individuals to be honest and vulnerable, thereby allowing true intimacy to emerge."

Clove - The oil of Boundaries

> "Clove supports individuals in letting go of victim mentality. Victims feel overly influenced by other people and outside circumstances. They perceive themselves as powerless to change their life situations. Clove assists individuals in letting go of patterns of self-betrayal and codependency by reconnecting them with their personal integrity."

Geranium - The oil of love and trust

"Geranium encourages emotional honesty, love and for-giveness. It fosters receptivity to human love and connection. Geranium aids in healing the broken heart."

Peppermint - The oil of a buoyant heart

"Peppermint brings joy and buoyancy to the heart and soul. It invigorates body, mind, and spirit and reminds individuals that life can be happy."

For these oils, I combined them (except the peppermint I save that for the end of the session to be applied neat to the spine) in a carrier oil and applied them to the areas of concentration on the body. Cinnamon and Clove oil are both hot! Use sparingly and it is wise to do a skin test on your subject before you begin. Use a few drops of the essential oils that have already been diluted in a carrier oil on a part of the body that isn't likely to be too much a bother if a negative reaction occurs. For example, I would choose my forearm to rub the oil in and make sure I haven't used too much of the hot oils. In general, one drop of cinnamon and clove in on ounce of olive oil (or your preferred carrier oil) isn't going to cause a problem. Be wise. Use your discretion. For my sessions I would combine all three oils into the carrier oil. Geranium is super strong, surprisingly so. I always use my diffuser but don't necessarily use one of the oils I had suggested for the specific sessions in it, something citrusy works well, uplifting! For your sessions, use what feels right to you.

Session Direction

Okay. Session 2. Let's do this. I'm so glad you're here!

For this session I want to realize feeling good. Let the focus revolve around the protective and supportive aspects of Psalm 91. He takes care of us. We are intending to cause the person to feel loving support through caring for the spine which is the flag pole of support for the body.

Jesus said, "According to your faith be it unto you."

Buddha said, "The mind is everything, what you think you become."

As we prepare to go into session set the intention of loving and supporting one's own self. I imagine myself to be a rechargeable battery. The way for me to get more juice once I'm drained is to plug into Jesus! I will stand alone before God one day. I alone am responsible for getting my God juice to be fully charged that I may feel good to charge fully! He has made a way.

Again I say, we are working together today to feel good.

Let your person lay face down covered by the sheet. To begin let's do a pelvic rock. Practitioner will place one hand over the sheet on the sacrum. Press down and move the hips back and forth in a gentle rocking motion. This feels really good and is relaxing. Do this rocking motion for a period of time that is meaningful for your particular session. Let your friend relax.

Okay, that was wonderful. Now it's time to pull the sheet down to the hips. Apply oil to the back. I like a lot of oil, not everybody does. The goal is to be able to glide the hands over the skin easily. This is a bit of an awkward position for the giver so make it work for you. You want to place both hands just below the waist one on each side of the spine, apply pressure and press up through the shoulder blades and gliding off at the shoulders. Do this three times nice and slow and easy.

Now we are ready to talk to the vertebrae and nerve structures within.

Reapply your massage oil as needed.

Beginning approximately at the top of the coccyx lay the hands flat on the back one hand on each side of the spine with the thumbs overlapping about a fingernail length. Now using the fingers for support lift the palms so the thumbs have mobility and move all the way up the spine to the base of the neck. Use the thumbs conversely to 'smooth out' the vertebrae, so to speak. Just applying some light pressure in upward and slightly outward strokes. Just one time up all the way to the base of the skull. Concentrate on being thorough.

Once completed, bring focus to the middle of the back beginning approximately at the thoracic vertebrae.

We will endeavor to touch each vertebrae individually in the thoracic and cervical spine. We want to clean and bless them as well as give them an intentional word of support. The thoracic spine, or middle to upper back, provides vital internal organs within the ribcage stability. It's made to hold fast. We want to provide this area of our bodies, designed to hang on, with a safe opportunity to release. This is a relaxing time. A time to slowly move from the middle of the spine up to the base of the skull. The idea is to open each vertebrae individually and clear it of any emotions or ideas associated with anger or bitterness about not being loved and protected properly. Then to speak love and health into it.

Does it seem ridiculous to believe this activity can make a difference? Is believing God and declaring His Word coupled with natural remedies really so different from putting one's faith in western medicine? This exercise has no side effects, neither do essential oils or faith in God's Word. They may however produce unthought of blessings. Whereas no one ever hears of surgeries or pharmaceuticals producing surprising benefits. It's commonly the opposite. Some new malady rears up to join the original issue. I'm not trying to say all western medicine and pharmaceuticals are evil. If I break a leg bone I'm hopping as fast as I can to the nearest emergency room. I'm just saying, it all takes faith. Give taking Jesus at His Word a chance.

If you run your fingers lightly up the spine you will usually feel the lumps of the vertebrae. Find the middle lump. Lightly, but enough pressure to feel, use your thumbs to open the vertebrae by placing the thumbs side by side over the area then dragging them out. I would just do three quick drags and consider the area open. With the vertebrae open, just as if you had a dishcloth and were wiping the counter clean, use your hand to wipe clear the vertebrae. Then use the middle and ring fingers to draw a circle around that area. While making the small circle, use your words to bless this vertebrae and plant a seed of love. A seed of what? Hope? Strength? Power? Courage? You can agree upon a list before hand or use music and sing over the spine. Your session your choice. After you've planted your circle seed now use all four fingers and press down over vertebrae sealing it back closed. Move to the next vertebrae. Do this up to the skull for each vertebrae.

Once finished take your peppermint oil and apply it neat, five to seven drops, over the spine. Rub this in so the essential oil soaks into the skin. Now cover your person back up and perhaps add a heavy blanket for comfort and warmth. Peppermint is cooling…

Move to the feet and finish with a beautiful foot massage for pleasure and relaxation.

Session 2 finished. Give yourself another week or two then move to session 3.

SESSION 3

Goal: Reconnecting the Reproductive System with Pleasure

Scripture Focus: Psalm 16

Suggested Oils:

Thyme - The oil of Releasing and Forgiving

> "Thyme is one of the most powerful cleansers of the emotional body and assists in addressing trapped feelings which have been buried for a long time. It reaches deep within the body and soul, searching for unresolved negativity. Thyme teaches that it's time to let go and move forward. As individuals forgive, they free themselves from emotional bondage."

Arborvitae: The oil of Divine Grace

> "Arborvitae assists individuals who believe or act like all progress must be made through struggle and solitary effort. It invites individuals to live with peace and joy by trusting in the abundant flow of divine grace."

Wild Orange - The oil of Abundance

"Wild Orange addresses a wide variety of emotional issues. It inspires abundance, fosters creativity, and supports a positive mood. Wild Orange also reconnects individuals with their inner child and brings spontaneity, fun, joy and playfulness into one's life."

Session Direction

Welcome to Session 3, my loves.

Remember Isaiah 61. Sometimes it's easy to believe the marring is eternal. So what's the use? Those are lies from hell though. We mustn't believe these thoughts generated from feeling bad about ourselves. It is true we feel bad. But bad feelings don't produce truth absolutely. So we look at what God says. Isaiah 61: 4 'He will rebuild the ancient ruins', our ruins aren't even ancient; seems like a fresh ruin would be easier to rebuild than one that's been long laid to waste.

Today we will look. Look at a place that, if our bodies really are temples, then this is the holy of holies. Who so dare enter ought to have a rope tied around their ankle in case they are found unworthy and be struck dead, then their grim carcass may be drug away. A veil exists as a warning and protection. It just isn't fair we must do this type of healing and draw back the veil in this way. But here we are. We are Ladies, helping each other, in a secret place 'shhh, proceed with reverence.' We are valiant! I just checked my thesaurus for 'valiant' and I like what it lists; Fearless. Gallant. Gutsy. Indomitable. Intrepid. Noble. Strong-willed. Vigorous.

110

Perversion hit me with its best shot. But I will not stay down. I will come back with a flaming sword. So, you might want to start running Perversion. Me and my Gutsy Gals are gunnin' for ya. Along with Jesus Christ. He is The One who makes our swords certain and effective!

Proceed with the tape exercise, My Gallant Friend. I believe in you and love you, and believe God is moving with loving-kindness on your behalf—even now, as I write this, He is making a way for you. Precious, Beautiful, Darling you!

The Tape Exercise

Before session three begins, there is need of both discussion and boundaries. This session endeavors to move the energy and memories of the genitals.

Our bodies are designed by God to feel and want pleasure. Many would argue the greatest transports of ecstasy and pleasure are to be found in the sex act. There are all kinds of pleasures out there—isn't it wonderful! The pleasure that comes from loving and being loved has such powerful magic that new life springs forth from its operations. Literally, a new life in the form of a baby person. One of God's greatest gifts to us, a child born out of pleasure and love.

Another one of God's greatest gifts is freewill. He has given each one of us the right to choose to believe and love Him and live the beautiful bountiful life He intends for us. Or, we may choose to disbelieve and reject Him and endeavor to follow our own path. In His goodness, He has set up the physical world to operate regardless of the type of association we choose to involve ourselves with Him. That is love! Therefore, the physical act of sex may still produce a child even if there is no love involved. Sometimes, even the violence of violation may produce a child. (Abortion is a topic I'm willing to discuss. If this has been something you've chosen, allow me to extend my deepest and most sincere condolences for your loss. God is able to make this situation benign. Remember He can make everything work together for the good of those who love Him (Romans 8:28). He wants to. There is more to say, but not here. Reach out to me. {cora@gutsandvictory.com}) As well, even though we may hate what is happening to us, our bodies may respond favorably to the physical manipulation of parts. In other words, our bodies, being made by God to function in response to certain stimulation, enjoy being touched. What am I saying? We liked being molested or raped? Certainly not! But, out bodies, none the less, may have felt the pleasure of stimulation. Even though it was 1000% nonconsensual, my body sometimes said, "Oh yeah, I like this."

Betrayed by my own body!

Part of me liked and wanted the pleasure that was a proper functioning of the body. My heart and mind hated the circumstances. That was an appropriate, rational, and emotional response. Because I was powerless to stop the interactions, myself, somehow, decided to stop my responses. I made a judgement that feeling good was bad. My mind and heart and spirit and soul set out to condemn feeling good in my body. Without understanding how or really why, as a child, I shut down my ability to have good sensuous feelings in response to stimulus. Learning how to restart them has been complex. Learning how to restart the good feelings is also disturbing because I needed to go back to the place where I stopped them. All emotions and visions in my mind surrounding that circumstance are enough misery to kill a horse. Who wants to admit to feeling good in these abusive scenarios? Nobody.

Laying all the garbage aside, keeping my eyes on the goal of reconnecting my reproductive system with pleasure, I acknowledge my desire. For the purposes of this exercise, call the center of origin of pleasure my vagina. Use whatever word you are comfortable with.

For this last session, it is necessary to wear yoga pants or something similar. Take a length of duct tape, or several and place the tape over the area you do not want touched during the session. Bearing in mind, for part of the session the legs fall open and the inner thigh is massaged. This is to provide a boundary and a feeling of safety while in a vulnerable spot.

For the subject, applying the tape is a special time to bring attention, awareness, compassion, forgiveness, and intentions to your private area. This area has been touched by evil. Time to cancel that touch and erase the ugly memories and emotions that may be hidden there. Create a new sensation, a new memory, a new response. Give yourself permission to feel good without guilt. Forgive your body. Give yourself understanding and acceptance. Forget the haters. Forget what is behind and strain towards what is ahead. Creating the good you want in your heart for your life.

The Practitioner will wait patiently for the Subject to finish with her tape exercise. While the tape exercise is going on the Practitioner may be about the business of setting up the space for this last session.

Priscilla Kapel, in her book, *The Body says Yes,* says, "We speak of 'legitimate' and 'ethical' massage as being non-sexual. In one sense, this is so, and in another it is an oversimplification. Non-sexual massage does carry a certain sexual charge for a great many people. All touching awakens feelings. If touching has been associated only with sex, all massage will be experienced as primarily sexual, regardless of the intent of the therapist. If touching evokes anxiety, the most tender massage will reach into that fear. After enough bodywork, these limitations and fears begin to change. Massage can awaken an appreciation for sensory pleasure which is not sexual, and can form positive associations with touching by opening trust in a fearful touch-deprived person. Our concern is not so much to address those issues as it is to open up the aliveness and streaming in the body."

We want to retrain this area to be 'alive' and 'awake' and receptive to loving, positive, consensual touch. Not all touch in this area need be sexual. My son came forth from this area and as a baby and small toddler, he is constantly between my legs jumping on me, laying on me, hugging me, grabbing me so he can steady himself. Our concern, as Priscilla Kapel eloquently states, is to 'open up the aliveness and streaming in the body.' What is streaming? I think it is positive motion and flow of oxygen, blood, and experience.

To this end when your person is ready, have her to lay on her back. [This session doesn't require a sheet because she is fully clothed in yoga gear. But she may still wish to have a blanket for covering up. It just feels good to be under blankies sometimes.] You will begin with a foot massage. Focusing on one foot at a time. Then to acquaint the legs with your kind touch, you will move up one leg, starting at the ankle, using both hands to hold the ankle and gently squeeze. Then move up a half an inch and gently squeeze. Move up the leg this way to the middle of the thigh then flatten both hands on the thigh, apply pressure and do a long gliding stroke off to the outer side of the leg and up the hip to the waist. Do this for both legs. Now we are ready to take pillows or blankets that have been rolled up and place them next to the outer thigh. Have your person bring her knees up so that her feet are flat on the ground. Have her legs fall open, landing on the pillows or blankets. These should be supporting her legs so the gravitational weight on her leg isn't pulling. It may take some adjusting to get the legs comfortably supported so they may lay open in butterfly position. Now the practitioner will sit close to the legs and, if beginning with the left leg, the practitioner will place her right hand on the left knee. Using her left hand, she will place her hand on the inside of the knee. Then with gentle gliding strokes, move her hand down the inner thigh—stopping before reaching the bending place and definitely keeping a measurable space away from the tape. Then just circle back up the leg to the knee. Take all pressure off when bringing the hand back up to the knee but maintain contact, and in this way continue for a period of time that is meaningful for your session. At this point, your person may still be flat of her back or may have requested to sit up being propped and supported with pillows. These are beautiful moments—just allowing our bodies to be touched in intimacy and safety. This is a good time to pray for your person's ability to let go of past yucky stuff, for her to go forward courageously, and for a more complete healing in this area, as well as increased circulation and improved muscle tone. Next, place the left hand on the knee and use the right hand to rub the hip. Circular motions with a pressure that is nice and comfortable for you both will do. Switch sides and repeat.

Once finished let the legs go back to laying straight out or whatever feels most comfortable. The practitioner may then move to the head of the subject and proceed with the forehead pull to finish off session 3.

And that's a wrap, kids.

Final thoughts and farewell

After your sessions be sure to give yourself extra grace and use your journal. Drink your water; it flushes toxins!

I feel like I'm saying 'Goodbye'. But it isn't true. I'm saying 'Farewell, for now.'

I hope this was helpful for you. More than that, life changing!

This is a beginning spot. I sometimes get to a place where I think I've made it. It feels like I'm walking on water for a few weeks then something surfaces. But I don't think this is unique to 'violated' people. We are all on a journey through this life and if we want to grow and be our best selves then we will learn and grow and make mistakes all the way through.

I have a list of resources that helped me on my website gutsandvictory.com

I hope to hear from you. In this life or the next.

ABOUT
KHARIS PUBLISHING

KHARIS PUBLISHING is an independent, traditional publishing house with a core mission to publish impactful books, and channel proceeds into establishing mini-libraries or resource centers for orphanages in developing countries, so these kids will learn to read, dream, and grow. Every time you purchase a book from Kharis Publishing or partner as an author, you are helping give these kids an amazing opportunity to read, dream, and grow. Kharis Publishing is an imprint of Kharis Media LLC. Learn more at **https://www.kharispublishing.com**.

www.ingramcontent.com/pod-product-compliance
Lightning Source LLC
Chambersburg PA
CBHW062101270326
41931CB00013B/3170